ALPHA DOCS

ALPHA DOCS

THE MAKING OF A CARDIOLOGIST

Daniel Muñoz, M.D.,
and James M. Dale

RANDOM HOUSE

NEW YORK

Alpha Docs is a work of nonfiction.
Some names and identifying details have been changed.

Published in the United States by Random House,
an imprint and division of Penguin Random House LLC,
New York.

RANDOM HOUSE and the HOUSE colophon are registered
trademarks of Penguin Random House LLC.

LIBRARY OF CONGRESS CATALOGING-IN-PUBLICATION DATA
Muñoz, Daniel, author.
Alpha docs : the making of a cardiologist / Daniel Muñoz, M.D., and
James M. Dale.
p. ; cm.
ISBN 978-1-4000-6887-6 (alk. paper) — ISBN 978-1-58836-953-6 (eBook)
I. Dale, James M., author. II. Title.
[DNLM: 1. Muñoz, Daniel. 2. Johns Hopkins Cardiovascular Fellows
Training Program. 3. Cardiology—education—Maryland—Personal
Narratives. 4. Fellowships and Scholarships—Maryland—
Personal Narratives. 5. Internship and Residency—
Maryland—Personal Narratives. WG 18]
RC682
616.1'20023—dc23
2014043542

Printed in the United States of America on acid-free paper

www.atrandom.com

2 4 6 8 9 7 5 3 1

FIRST EDITION

Book design by Christopher M. Zucker

To Olivia, Lucas, and their superhero
mother

—Daniel Muñoz

To Ellen, as usual, as always

—James M. Dale

A Note from the Authors

The stories depicted in this book are based on, or derived from, real-world medical situations. In order to protect the privacy of patients and families, names, personal and medical details, and other identifying characteristics have been changed. The names of attending doctors have been changed to the first or middle names of U.S. presidents. Other medical personnel names and details have also been changed.

Contents

INTRODUCTION: *A Life-Changing Event*   xi

1. CARDIOVASCULAR FELLOWSHIP   3
The Match Process with a Twist

2. ROTATION: CARDIAC CONSULTATION   9
Suddenly, I'm a Cardiologist

3. ROTATION: NUCLEAR MEDICINE, PART I   18
Anything "Nuclear" Sounds Impressive

4. DISTANCE AND PERSPECTIVE   26
Sometimes You Have to Get Away from
Medicine to See It Clearly

5. FELLOWS' CASE CONFERENCE   31
My Turn

6. ROTATION: PREVENTIVE CARDIOLOGY, PART I   39
Patient, Heal Thyself

7. ROTATION: HEART FAILURE AND HEART
TRANSPLANTATION, PART I   51
Who Gets a Heart, Who Doesn't

8. ROTATION: CARDIAC INTENSIVE CARE UNIT, PART I   72
The Other Hopkins

9. **ROTATION: ELECTROPHYSIOLOGY**   97
   Circuit Board of the Heart

10. **ROTATION: NUCLEAR MEDICINE, PART II**   114
   A Christmas Present

11. **ROTATION: CARDIAC INTENSIVE CARE UNIT, PART II**   123
   There's No Such Thing as "Routine"

12. **ROTATION: HEART FAILURE AND HEART TRANSPLANTATION, PART II**   148
   As a Sort-of Veteran

13. **ROTATION: ECHOCARDIOGRAPHY, PART I**   172
   Little Pictures in a Quiet, Dark Room

14. **COSTA RICA**   179
   Reflections on What I'll Be When I Grow Up

15. **ROTATION: ECHOCARDIOGRAPHY, PART II**   183
   I Get to Drive

16. **ROTATION: CARDIAC CATHETERIZATION— INTERVENTIONAL CARDIOLOGY**   191
   The Closest We Get to Being Surgeons

17. **WEEKEND COVERAGE**   202
   A Virtual Two-Day Rotation

18. **ROTATION: PREVENTIVE CARDIOLOGY, PART II**   212
   Working with the Guru

19. **365 DAYS A FELLOW**   219
   What I Learned

EPILOGUE: *What Kind of Heart Doctor Will I Be?*   223

Acknowledgments   229

Introduction

A LIFE-CHANGING EVENT

East Baltimore in July, and the temperature and humidity are an identical, unbearable ninety-eight. It wasn't raining, but walking one block left you soaked. I walked three. That was my route within the invisible Johns Hopkins safety zone, the world's biomed fortress, surrounded by lead-painted welfare housing and occasional crack dens. By the time I stepped into the outpatient entrance, my shirt was like a second skin. A blast of AC turns the perspiration to a chill as I enter the underground tunnel that leads to the main hospital, content to be out of the heat for the next thirty hours. Nothing about this night seems different from any of the others I've spent as the internal medicine resident on the cardiac intensive care unit (CICU) rotation—but then, life-changing moments rarely come with advance warning.

In the CICU, the attending doctor leads the team—a cardiology Fellow and a small squad of residents that includes me—through rounds, patient by patient, checking charts and meds. The attending fires questions like the lightning round of a game show; we spit back answers and then move on to the next bed. When we finish, the attending glances outside, through a window steamed with sweat, and casually says, "This is the kind of weather that can kill people."

He's right. Not far from the hospital, at 6:00 p.m., a man named Randy is walking through Patterson Park in East Baltimore. In the daytime, Patterson is still just a park, full of kids on bicycles, joggers, and softball teams. But a few hours later, darkness transforms it into an open-air drug market, where people such as Randy can buy a small packet of coke, their little nightly jolt. Out of a job and with nowhere else to be, Randy lights a cigarette and waits for night to fall.

Randy is thirty-nine, but an overweight, dissipated thirty-nine. Even the short walk from the southeast corner of the park to the crisscross at its center has exhausted him. He sits down on a splintered green bench and waits for the fatigue to go away, but it doesn't. His chest feels strangely heavy, as if something were sitting on his rib cage. Even when Randy stretches out on the bench, the unfamiliar pressure refuses to let up.

An old woman walks by, a park regular who pushes a stroller filled with empty bottles and cans, but no baby. Seeing Randy, she stops and asks, "You okay?" He doesn't answer. "You need help?" He tries to shake his head, but it won't move. The woman starts to walk away, then turns back. "Want me to call an ambulance?" Hearing Randy's faintly whispered "Yeah," the elderly lady fishes a flip phone out of her collection of bottles and cans, and dials 911.

When the EMTs find Randy on the bench, they ask him his age, name, and pain level; check his vital signs; then roll him onto a gurney and into the ambulance. After putting an oxygen mask on Randy and hooking him up to an IV, the medics phone ahead to Johns Hopkins with the data: time, 6:47 p.m.; thirty-nine-year-old male with substernal chest pain; 10 out of 10 on pain scale; nauseous; likely MI (myocardial infarction) according to the electrocardiogram (EKG) in the ambulance, eight to ten minutes from the emergency room (ER).

The call from ambulance to hospital is a trigger, alerting each of the appropriate hospital care units to be ready. Even though Randy is a heavy-smoking, obese, habitual drug user without a job, having a life-threatening emergency in the locale of East Baltimore means one thing: He is headed to Johns Hopkins, one of the top-ranked hospitals in the United States. Unlucky Randy has lucked out on this one thing.

The Hopkins ER—a contradiction of rusty steam pipes and chirping digital monitors—has a bed slot ready. By the time the ambulance team bashes the swinging doors open with the gurney, another team is waiting for the handoff. An ER nurse hooks Randy up to the twelve leads (sensors) for the EKG, which will measure the rhythm and strength of his heartbeat. Another nurse draws blood to check whether elevated enzyme and protein levels are leaking into Randy's bloodstream. Definitive lab results will take ninety minutes— minutes that Randy doesn't have. The nurses give Randy aspirin, slip a nitroglycerin tablet under his tongue, and connect his IV to a cocktail of morphine and heparin, to help the pain and thin his blood. Meanwhile, Randy pants. He can't seem to catch his breath. The weight on his chest is relentless.

The attending emergency room doctor and his resident read the jagged lines on Randy's EKG, looking for "STEMI," an elevation in the ST segment of the EKG that indicates MI. Although Randy's EKG is ambiguous, it is abnormal enough to kick off a series of rehearsed responses: The STEMI code is sent to the pagers carried by both the cardiac catheterization team and the cardiac intensive care unit doctors, and the EKG printout is faxed up to my team in the CICU on the fifth floor. My CICU Fellow and I each see the EKG and draw the likely conclusion: This heart tissue may be dying. This is a significant moment for me: Perhaps for the first time, I think I know what this is. And I know what to do. With no time to waste on extra conversation, he says, "Let's make sure," and nods toward the portable echocardiogram— the ultrasound machine. As I roll it into the elevator, I barely have time to register the significance of my personal moment of clarity.

After navigating a service elevator and three hallways, we arrive at Randy's bedside, to find his breathing even more labored. The pressure on his chest has increased from a box of bricks to a small elephant. Randy is in visible distress, and he is scared: "Doc, am I having a heart attack?" I look over at the CICU Fellow, who is so intent on the echo images that he doesn't seem to hear Randy. For now, all I can do is give Randy safe but impossible-to-follow advice: "Try to relax."

The evidence from the echocardiogram is undeniable. The anterior wall of his heart is barely moving, indicating that it is not getting enough blood. And if his heart wall is dying, then Randy might be next. Already his color is gone, his breathing shallower. We have, at most, two minutes to make our assessment. It takes seconds: One look and two nods, and the CICU Fellow gives the order: "Get him to the cath lab."

The head ER nurse asks Randy whom to notify of his condition. He mumbles, "Nobody." They put hospital forms in front of him, and he signs. That small act of signing his name was exhausting. "Am I gonna be all right?" he asks as his bed is wheeled onto the elevator to the catheterization lab.

The cath lab looks like "the future" in a science fiction movie: a blindingly bright, antiseptic, totally silent chamber. The CICU Fellow and I watch from a control room, shielded from the radiation that the fluoroscopic imaging generates. The cath team preps Randy and begins to snake a catheter into his femoral artery. The lab is kept at a constant sixty-eight degrees, but we can see that Randy, terrified and in pain, is soaked in perspiration.

Randy, covered in sterile drapes and monitoring equipment, is awake throughout, as the catheter travels into the femoral artery, against the tide of blood flow, into the iliac artery, up the aorta, past the aortic arch, to the juncture at the aortic valve where the arteries branch off the aorta to feed the heart. The team then injects a dye into the catheter to locate the occlusion. A camera registers the strong flow of the dye until it hits a blockage in Randy's left anterior descending artery (LAD). The width of the flow goes from a drinking straw to a strand of thread. This miniature dam, less than a centimeter in length, is why Randy is here.

The team snakes in the angioplasty line, a second catheter that remains small and flat until it reaches the critical spot, at which point it is inflated like a balloon to stretch open the blocked artery. After inflating the angioplasty line, the cath team injects more dye, this time to see if blood can flow through the opened section. For a moment, everyone holds their breath. Then the dye rushes through, followed by essential blood, nutrients, and oxygen. Seconds later, Randy relaxes and lets out a sigh of relief so immense that it seems to hover in the air. The elephant has rolled off his chest.

What Randy does not know is that the balloon is a temporary fix. He isn't out of the woods yet. A third catheter containing a stent (a small hollow cage, collapsed for transport) must be inserted and maneuvered to the spot opened by the balloon, then deployed to keep the artery open. The CICU Fellow and I track the video fluoroscopy as the dye is reshot through the catheter in what seems like slow motion, waiting to see if the stent worked, if the dye and the blood can now flow through. Practice and statistics say they will, but problems—misplacement, misreading, a tear, the unknown—can still arise. Two seconds. Randy could still reocclude his LAD. He could still end up with severe heart damage. Three seconds. He could still die. Four seconds . . .

At last, the dye flows through. There is a moment when the cath team, the CICU Fellow, and I all collectively exhale. No one, no matter how experienced, treats this as routine.

Now that Randy is in the clear, the team snaps back into action: It's time to clean up and get out. The three catheters are removed, but the sheath in Randy's groin remains in order to prevent his thinned blood from bleeding out. Randy is smiling as he is rolled out of the cath lab, down several corridors, and into a room in the cardiac intensive care unit. A team of nurses hooks him up to monitors and checks his vital signs. I tell him to try to relax, knowing that, this time, it isn't impossible-to-follow advice.

Leaving Randy, I grab a quick cup of coffee and sit alone,

taking the opportunity to gather my thoughts. It is 8:25 p.m. Everything from the EMT report through to the procedure and Randy's return to the CICU has happened in less than two hours. A thirty-nine-year-old, overweight, smoking, drug-using male had a heart attack. We had saved his life, at least for the moment. And I was part of it.

I stared at my hands, wondering what, ultimately, I would do with them. My education, my experience, my instincts, had played a critical role in saving a patient, but, at the same time, at a crucial moment, I had been an observer, behind the glass, watching others carry out the life-changing procedure. What did I want to do? Which side of the glass did I want to be on? Once again, I was faced with my recurring career multiple-choice test, starting with the serious options: (a) an internist, (b) a pulmonologist, (c) an oncologist, (d) a cardiologist. Usually, as the right answer eluded me, I would wander into the less serious: (e) a fireman, (f) a baseball player, or (g) an astronaut. But that night, as I thought back to how I'd watched the cath team at work, I could feel the answer beginning to form.

I returned to check on Randy. Now that he was in the CICU after successful emergency stenting, the challenge was to keep him healthy, hopefully for years, but critically for tonight. The heart doctors would start him on medications— a beta-blocker, blood thinners to inhibit clot-prone platelets from forming new blockages—a diet, a light exercise regimen, and a schedule of checkups.

Randy, still shaken by what had happened, promised to do exactly as we said. I asked questions about his life— parents, marriage, children. When he said he was married but it didn't work, he had a little girl but didn't see her, he had lost touch with family . . . it made me pause. Randy was alone, a drug user, a guy living on the fringe who had come in off the streets, and by the mere geography of where he had his heart incident, a fluke. Or was he? The more I probed, the more I realized how normal Randy was. He had traveled, done odd jobs as a cook, as a bartender, and on a fishing boat. He liked to listen to Orioles games on the radio, even though they almost never won. "They're bad. I love 'em 'cause they're bad." Randy was just another guy, with ups and downs and experiences that made him unique but hardly extraordinary.

Randy had his quirks. So did the sheiks, CEOs, politicians, and well-heeled royalty who often checked into Johns Hopkins. Whether they had wives or husbands or children or jobs or fame or drug habits, they all had bodies and flawed organs and hearts that could stop beating. It was chance that had brought Randy to Johns Hopkins, where he was able to get the best treatment available in the world.

For Randy, the night had been life-changing. It was also life-changing for me. I knew where I wanted to be: not watching but doing, on the side of the glass where I can help shape a patient's fate. I would be a cardiologist. I wasn't thinking about where I'd train or how long or under whom. I knew I was choosing a demanding path. But I knew I wanted to be a heart doctor.

*   *   *

Every year in the U.S., approximately 800,000 people die of cardiovascular-related disease. 720,000 have a heart attack; 620,000 for the first time and 295,000 recurrent. All told, an astonishing one-quarter of all Americans—over 80,000,000 people—live with or die from some form of cardiovascular disease.

—*American Heart Association, December 2013*

Then there are the heart doctors. According to "The Match" (The National Resident Matching Program), the official body that links doctors to training programs, a little over thirty thousand doctors apply for specialty residencies—pediatrics, radiology, neurology, general surgery, or internal medicine—each year. Only twenty-four thousand are chosen to be residents. In my year, of the sixty-five hundred residents who applied for an internal medicine subspecialty fellowship—gastroenterology, clinical oncology, hematology, cardiovascular disease—roughly forty-five hundred made the cut. In cardiology, one of the most selective subspecialties, success is often 50 percent at best. And at the most elite cardiology programs—Hopkins, Harvard, Columbia, Duke, Cleveland Clinic, Mayo Clinic, UCSF, Penn, and a few others—the odds are still tougher.

The Johns Hopkins Cardiovascular Disease Training Fellowship Program receives five hundred to seven hundred impeccably credentialed, impressive applications from all parts of the world, but only nine are "ranked to match." Only nine will receive training from some of the most brilliant, demanding cardiac practitioners and professors in the world.

In the course of the fellowship, they will learn to practice cardiology at its highest level. They will learn to search for elusive symptoms, and cure what resists cure. They will attempt heroic treatments, some of which succeed and some of which do not. They will face terrified families and bring them near miracles. They will face hopeful families and have to deliver devastating news. The experience will be an exhilarating, wrenching, breathtaking, brutal ordeal, at once ego-making and ego-breaking, heroic and humbling, part science and part art.

Their story is my story. I am one of the nine, a cardiology Fellow at Johns Hopkins. I am living it daily, rotation after rotation, patient after patient, family after family, diagnosing and treating patients, staying up all day and then all night, learning from mentors, some geniuses, some egomaniacs, struggling to save lives, and coming to terms with losing them. This is my real-time, real-life chronicle of what it means to become a heart doctor at an elite cardiology program in one of America's most renowned hospitals.

I had no idea how demanding it was going to be.

ALPHA DOCS

CARDIOVASCULAR FELLOWSHIP

The Match Process with a Twist

July, one year later. I'm standing outside Johns Hopkins again, at an hour when most people are heading home from work, about to begin the first rotation of my cardiovascular training. Each rotation is an immersion in a subspecialty. Most run four weeks, some two, some repeat with two segments. By the end of the fellowship, not only are you supposed to be educated and proficient in every area, but it's assumed that you'll know what kind of heart doctor you'd like to be. Will you go to work in interventional cardiology, with caths and stents? Will you end up reading stress test films in nuclear? Will you be in preventive, changing patient lifestyles, or working in the more dramatic area of transplant? Fellowship is a countdown to yet another decision day.

Unlike residency, which is a form of group learning, fellowship builds individual relationships, one Fellow working closely with one or two attendings on each rotation. And unlike residency, the other Fellows aren't likely to become our friends and surrogate family. We'll see one another only occasionally, in meetings, in hallways, at a case conference.

Still, we'd all briefly met and sized one another up yesterday, during the cardiology fellowship orientation. Clasping our packets of information about the basics of parking, health insurance, campus map, phone numbers—papers we'll likely never look at again—we had smiled and shared small chuckles about our contracts. These papers state our salaries, benefits, et cetera, and we're supposed to read and sign them. The fact is, there's no reason to. We've been winnowed from thousands to hundreds to nine. We all want to be Hopkins cardiologists. We've already signed up for this deal.

Rotation order is mostly random, but sometimes the faculty can change it up and make judgment calls. I'm starting with cardiology consults, considered one of the most demanding rotations of all. I won't have total medical responsibility for any of the patients, but I will have cardiac responsibility for patients whose issues can range from a routine inquiry on the dosage of a beta-blocker to a postsurgical weekend jock who goes into cardiac arrest in recovery. I'm pretty sure I got consults first because of a Hopkins prejudice—that a Hopkins-trained resident is more ready for trial by fire. We know our way around the hospital, and that's no small thing whether you're looking for the SICU (surgical intensive care unit) or a bathroom. Other than that, the biggest difference between me today and me two days ago as a senior resident is the word *Fellow* stitched above my name on my white coat.

I look up at the dome on the roof of the old hospital building, the icon that says, "This is Hopkins—the best," and think back on how I got here. I'm almost thirty years old, pursuing a career that often feels like a distant mirage: No matter how close I get, it always seems a little further away, and when I haven't slept for thirty-six hours, I wonder if my profession will ever start or if I'll forever be "in training." I went to Princeton for four years, Johns Hopkins Medical School for four years, interrupted by a year at Harvard for a master's in public administration, then a Hopkins residency in internal medicine for three years, and now a Hopkins cardiovascular fellowship for three or four more years. Plenty of doctors choose not to do a fellowship in a subspecialty. After years of training, and after seeing their peers rise through the ranks in nonmedical professions, they want to get started. Many of my friends have earned hundreds of thousands of dollars in the time I've run up loans for nearly as much. But, after the impact on me of the events with Randy, I knew I wanted to keep going, to extend my training and pursue a fellowship in cardiology.

That meant entering the annual "match" last year. The match is the computer-assisted mating dance, which narrows applicant pools to on-site interviews before assessing the ranked preferences of the final applicants and the programs. Acceptance is based on a combination of clinical work during residency, evaluations of residency attending staff, research the candidate may have done, and a personal statement, the closest thing to a wild card or tiebreaker—

what you've done that could set you apart from the hundreds of overachievers vying for the same few slots.

There is something called the rule of 10 in selection processes. It maintains that being chosen gets exponentially harder each time you take another step up the ladder, whether it's from the county beauty pageant to the state pageant, or from a high school team to Division I. If getting into the most selective colleges, on a 1-to-10 scale, is 10, then getting into the best graduate or medical schools is 10×10, and getting into the best residency is 10×100, and getting into the most selective fellowship is $10 \times 1,000$, or 1 in 10,000.

I still remember my interview day at Hopkins. After all the applicants were treated to an ironically high-cholesterol breakfast spread, Dr. Fitzgerald—the head of the program—walked in. He not only knew all of our names and where we went to school, but he created a story, in one endless sentence, weaving in our individual interests, hometowns, talents, siblings, foibles, everything. "Sara, we're glad you were able to travel all the way from Barcelona, especially since you'd probably rather be helicopter-skiing in the Andes, which Amit could appreciate, having just returned from Pakistan's K-2 summit, which he first climbed as an undergrad at Oxford, coincidentally where Maya studied Old English poetry before switching to premed (our gain, their loss), and the same could be said about Dan since he's divided his time between medicine and Washington health policy for the past three years, a far cry from Raj, who locked himself in a room to finish a book about . . ."

It was more than an entertaining performance or a stroking of our young egos. It also sent a message: "We know you. We put time into this because we will put time into you. Of all the candidates, we think you will become the best cardiologists if you come to Johns Hopkins."

After a tour of the facility came the individual interviews with faculty members, each a medical version of a police interrogation. Where'd you grow up? Play sports? Travel? Where'd you go to college? I see you had a rocky year first year of med school. What happened? Too demanding? Why do you want to be a cardiologist? Why Hopkins? What makes you think you can make it here?

I went on nine of those tours and interviews: Johns Hopkins, Brigham and Women's Hospital (Harvard), University of California at San Francisco, Duke, Northwestern, Columbia, Penn, University of Virginia, University of Maryland. Then I submitted my order of preference to The Match process and the institutions did likewise—and where the two rankings intersect, the matches would be made . . . all very objectively, very algorithmically.

But not always. Sometimes, institutions can unofficially make direct human contact with candidates to signal their feelings.

I had one of those conversations when the same Dr. Fitzgerald asked me to stop by his office. One of his tasks was to target two or three Hopkins residents to stay at Hopkins for their cardiology fellowships. He was very up front with me: "Dan, you're at the top of our list for the cardiology fellowship program." I was a little stunned. I'd hoped to match with Hopkins, but "the top of the list"? It wasn't easy to tell him I'd mentally ranked Hopkins and Harvard in a tie for first place, but I did. He said he respected my thinking, told me to take my time and then decide. In other words, come to Hopkins.

A couple of days later, I got virtually the same call from Harvard. Choosing between these two was a great problem to have, but not one I could share. Hopkins? Harvard? No one would sympathize. In the end, I made a rational-emotional decision. I'd chosen to become a cardiologist that day with Randy at Hopkins; Hopkins is where I'd see it through.

I called Dr. Fitzgerald and told him. He didn't seem surprised.

That was December. Now here I am.

I walk back inside. It's five o'clock. As of this moment, the system considers me a cardiologist. After all, I have a white coat that says so.

2

ROTATION: CARDIAC CONSULTATION

Suddenly, I'm a Cardiologist

The cardiac consult team is lead by the attending physicians, the senior faculty members responsible for all recommendations and treatments. As a Fellow, I will work with one attending for the first two weeks, and another for the second two weeks. The first is Dr. George, an Australian with an Outback Steakhouse accent, in his late fifties, soft-spoken, a down-to-earth doctor's doctor, reassuring to his patients and to me. The second is Dr. John, an older, hardened Hopkins veteran, who I've heard is a firm believer in the hands-off approach, which, for a Fellow, means you're left on your own. You'll get to carry the weight—but that might not be best for either the student or the patient.

In addition to the attendings, there's a medical student doing a fourth-year elective rotation. Ours is Joseph, a high-caliber med student who was raised in upstate New York.

He's from a large Italian family of academics, and we connect over our love of baseball. He's smart enough to assume responsibility when things get hectic. By all appearances, we're a very respectable team.

There's just one small thing: I don't know how to perform an echo (a cardiac ultrasound test), and without that skill, I'm not much use on the rotation. I was never taught in residency because it's not essential to a resident. Watching an echo being performed on Randy in the ER is as close as I've been. They're supposedly not hard to do; I just don't know how, and they're ordered day and night. During the day, the ultrasound team, led by a technician, takes the machine to a patient's bedside, administers the test, and the echo lab team interprets it. These daytime echoes are by and large routine. But after 5:00 p.m. today, when my consult rotation starts, until who knows when, there's no team, just me, the Fellow on call. And the middle of the night is when the nonroutine, emergency-type echoes seem to happen, and therefore fall to the cardiologists in training, such as me. So I really need to know how to do them.

I find the head of the echo lab, confess my ignorance, request a crash course, and ask for a pledge of confidentiality. She's sympathetic in a motherly, "This happens every year" way. I follow her down a hall to an oversize closet full of broken chairs, bed rails, bedpans, sheets, door handles, and IV stands. She uses the ultrasound cart to plow some of the detritus out of the way to create a work space, and closes the door. It's safe to say no one will come in, since no one has in years. For the next ninety minutes, she shows me how to do a basic echo, assessing for overall ventricular function and the presence of a pericardial effusion (fluid collection in the sac surrounding the heart, which, if severe, can be deadly). She takes me through the steps, over and over, until I've mastered Ultrasound for Dummies.

Now that I can do an ultrasound, the team is ready for prime time.

The unstated mandate of cardiology training is: Learn fast. We aren't technically on call all night, but the reality is that my pager beeps almost anytime, day or night. It can be a sixty-second query from a resident in surgery who needs cardiac-related recommendations for post-op care: Patient A just came out of gastric bypass surgery for obesity, and we need to know if there may be any adverse effects of administering fifty milligrams of atenolol, blood pressure medication. Or it can be a four-hour high-intensity drill: Patient B has developed severe hypotension—blood pressure drop—in the midst of bladder cancer surgery. What do we do? How do we do it? When? For the most part, I either know the answers or can come up with a strategy to arrive at them. When I'm sure, I make the call. When I'm not, I check with Dr. George. The key is knowing the difference.

This kind of pressure means that newly minted Fellows tend to share a dark humor: "Another good day. I didn't kill anyone." That humor turns out to be one of the few bonds among us, as we intersect in hallways, on breaks, or when two of us are seeing the same patient for different reasons.

A few days go by, and just when I start to think that consults isn't so daunting, I'm thrown into a situation that reminds me of the gravity of what we do. It's my second week on the rotation, and I'm brought in on the case of an eighty-one-year-old woman, Midge, who has come in for surgery to remove a tumor on her liver. The tumor turns out to be malignant, and she's slated to begin cancer treatment. But it's only after complex surgery when she's in the intensive care unit (ICU) that a routine electrocardiogram (EKG) reveals strain on her heart with mildly elevated cardiac enzyme levels. I'm being consulted because we need to figure out whether (a) the EKG and enzymes are evidence of an evolving heart blockage or (b) they're relatively predictable signs of stress following major surgery. The stakes are high because the two possible diagnoses indicate almost polar opposite treatments. Post-op stress means Midge should be watched carefully. Evolving coronary blockage means a series of steps, including an invasive procedure such as catheterization, and/or blood thinners, which carry their own risk for a person who has just had abdominal surgery—that is, bleeding. There isn't any yes/no test to determine the right conclusion. It's a judgment call. And it's up to my team to make it.

The basic issue is one of supply versus demand. Supply issues are what heart attacks are made of. An acute compromise of blood supply (coronary plaque rupture/clot) results in an urgent or emergent trip to the cath lab while blood thinners are administered, similar to what happened with Randy. Unless the supply is reestablished by angioplasty (opening the blocked artery), the heart muscle begins dying, meaning that, without intervention, the patient may also. On the other hand, an increase in myocardial demand (the heart muscle's need for oxygen and the blood's nutrients) can induce strain on the heart muscle, and sometimes result in heart cell death. The solution to this problem is different, since it involves relieving the stress, treating the infection, eliminating the dehydration, controlling the bleeding. In this case, you have to fix the underlying stressor.

In Midge's case, we need to figure out whether she is having a heart attack caused by plaque rupture and a new clot lodging in one of her coronary arteries, or is simply experiencing postoperative cardiac stress because of her surgery. Heart cells die when supply and demand don't agree. Figuring out why they're out of balance, and what to do, is part of the nuts and bolts of cardiology.

I spend a full hour going over Midge's chart. I question the surgical resident. I speak to the ICU nurses. And I attempt to assess her directly, although Midge can't talk because she's been intubated and is currently dependent on a mechanical ventilator. The resident introduces me to Midge's family as the cardiologist who will care for her heart while Midge recovers from surgery. It's a small untruth: There's no upside in telling nervous relatives you're only "studying" to be a cardiologist. I take my time to understand Midge's background, and ask her daughter and a family friend about Midge's level of physical mobility and about any previous heart problems. I learn that Midge leads an active lifestyle: She walks for forty-five minutes to an hour every day with her daughter, has no history of heart problems, and is an avid gardener.

I ask the surgical team to order an echo (done by the in-house tech). The ultrasound can reveal critical information about what region of Midge's heart might be injured. If Midge has a new blockage or clot resulting in a decreased blood supply, then a part of the heart wall wouldn't work as well and the ultrasound would indicate that. From that standpoint, her echo images are reassuring, showing the heart squeezing as it should. I also ask the surgical team to check cardiac enzyme levels every six hours, since a blockage or clot can also cause enzymes to leak into the bloodstream. A day later, the results come in: Midge's cardiac enzyme levels were mildly elevated but fortunately now seem to be trending down.

This news is good but not definitive, and the surgical resident needs a conclusion. I explain that I do not think Midge is having a heart attack, but rather is experiencing postoperative cardiac stress. For the time being, all we should do is keep a careful eye on Midge.

Over the next several days, the immediate evidence seems to confirm my judgment. It turns out that pneumonia was the likely stressor. When I visit Midge later, she is no longer hooked up to as many tubes and monitors and, now surrounded by her daughter and grandchildren, appears the image of a strong, resilient matriarch. Although Midge later develops other complications, which require two more trips to the operating room, her heart functions well under the strain. I had made the right call: Because she was never put on blood thinners—as she would have been if there had been a clot or blockage—she was able to have these surgeries without additional risk.

I survived my first real test. Unfortunately, Midge has a particularly awful form of liver cancer. Statistics say she has only eighteen to twenty-four months to live. Even though I made the right call, and even though we fixed the heart problem, we cannot fix the cancer. It's not a victory—just a delay.

My attending, Dr. George, is a reassuring, hands-on mentor, who guides me through each case and outcome, including this one, showing me what I did right and what could have been done better. He's always there with the safety net, just in case. Working with Dr. George, I feel as if I'm doing well, although I see so little of the other Fellows that I have no point of comparison (as is usual in fellowship).

Weeks three and four are another story. My new attending is Dr. John, a sharp contrast to Dr. George; his approach is to let me find my way. I'm on my own, almost being dared to fail. Over the next two weeks, I see patients throughout all parts of the hospital—as many as six or eight a day. Each time my pager beeps, I run a mental drill of what I will do: Take a deep breath, clear my mind, and then call the doctor back (urologist, surgeon, gynecologist, ENT [ear, nose, and throat] specialist). I listen to the case, ask key questions, and examine the patient. Then I process all the information and determine the next steps in diagnosis and/or treatment. But before implementing a plan, I call Dr. John, who listens to my summary as if he were preoccupied with something else, waits for my assessment, then grunts "Uh-huh," and hangs up. His near silence is his form of approval. Working with Dr. John is cardiology without training wheels.

Case after case after case: I'm on a roll. A woman coming out of labor with a fast heart rate. A young man with a drop in blood pressure after a bowel resection. Several elderly patients with swelling that might be due to congestive heart failure. The closest Dr. John comes to "input" is one case in which I conclude that the patient's post-op arrhythmias warranted a transfer to the cardiac intensive care unit. This time, I'm surprised to hear him say "You sure?" I double-check the data and realize that I *am* sure, and go ahead with the transfer.

It's my last week on cardiology consults when I am called by the trauma surgery team to see a fifty-two-year-old man, Mr. Rosen, who has been brought in by ambulance following a car accident. After his lacerations are cleaned, Mr. Rosen reports feeling chest pain. His EKG looks normal, apart from a couple of small vagaries. The trauma team is worried about acute coronary syndrome, which is a catchall for clinical symptoms of acute myocardial ischemia (insufficient blood supply to the heart), which can come in varying degrees of severity.

On my way to the ER, I call Dr. John with a run-through of the case. He says, "Tell me how it goes afterward." He doesn't ask anything more about the patient's condition. He doesn't ask for my take on the situation. He doesn't tell me to call if I have a question. He just assumes I'll know what to do . . . or I'll call if I need him.

In the ER, I check on Mr. Rosen's electrocardiogram. It appears to be normal, which is reassuring—the "vagaries" don't mean anything unless there are other indicators. I examine Mr. Rosen and see no signs of congestive heart failure, no fluid backing up into his lungs.

What he does have is profound wheezing, very labored breathing. I look at his X ray with the surgeons: no punctured lung, no obvious fractures, no evidence of pneumonia. The one notable finding is the degree to which his lungs are hyperinflated (expanded), a telltale sign of a smoker's lungs or COPD (chronic obstructive pulmonary disease), most commonly known as emphysema. I decide to administer steroids and a series of nebulizer breathing treatments. Mr. Rosen relaxes, and his breathing and chest pain get better. I report this to Dr. John. He grunts his "Uh-huh."

I did this cardiac consult solo, and it went fine: It turned out that Mr. Rosen's possible angina was just a breathing issue related to smoking. The Dr. John method worked. That night I find myself thinking about which attending's style is better—hands-on or hands-off. The answers, for patients or for young doctors, are almost diametrically opposite. Before this rotation, I would have said the hands-on method is better, the safety net for patients being obvious. But then doctors such as me would never learn to do what we have to do. And now that I've succeeded without a net, I realize that maybe a little fear is a good thing. For learning, anyway.

Perhaps the net was there all along—I just didn't see it. And because I didn't see it, I learned to rely on myself, to trust my judgment even when Dr. John second-guessed me. Maybe Dr. John knew that I could push myself further and handle the pressure. Maybe. But doesn't a patient deserve more than a young cardiology Fellow hoping that he or she has made the right call? It's a trade-off, teaching versus treating. The answer is clear. You have to teach . . . but, as popularly paraphrased from the Hippocratic oath, *first, do no harm.*

Okay, I've made it through cardiac consults—an onslaught of cases, questions, diagnoses, and decisions, almost eight weeks of hours packed into four—a total immersion. Still, I am no closer to knowing what kind of cardiologist I will be, but, I rationalize, this is only the first rotation. And I'm learning some key lessons—how to perform an ultrasound, to "consult" on what may or may not be cardiac issues and know the difference, to trust my instincts a little more each day, and, as in the case of Midge, accept that even when we win a heart battle, sometimes another illness trumps and we lose the war.

3

ROTATION: NUCLEAR MEDICINE, PART I

Anything "Nuclear" Sounds Impressive

My next rotation is in nuclear medicine, which sounds impressive but just means reading stress tests. And even "stress tests" sounds more impressive than the reality: putting people on treadmills to see how fast and far they can go without pain. These tests are prescribed for patients who might have abnormal blood supply (ischemic heart disease) or who need a prognosis for recovery from a heart attack (myocardial infarction). For the Fellows, stress testing means less stress compared to other rotations, especially after four weeks of cardiology consults. Whereas cardiology consults can be eighty-hour weeks, nuclear weeks are technically forty hours, with the actual work time a fraction of that. Again, the rotation order is supposed to be random, but the ups and downs seem planned. They run us until we drop. They let us recover. Then they run us again.

The skills that nuclear hones are fundamental to cardiac care and clinical decision making. We're not observing the administration of the stress tests; we're learning to read the results. Although we're welcome to watch the actual test performance, there's not much to see that we haven't seen as med students or residents—sweaty, panting patients on a treadmill and, once in a while, chest pain that stops the test.

So three afternoons a week, we sit in the back offices, overseen by nuclear attending staff, as the results come in from the Hopkins main downtown hospital and from all the outlying Hopkins clinics around the city. We read five to ten studies on Mondays, Tuesdays, and Thursday, from four in the afternoon until six or seven. All told, an entire week of nuclear is eight to ten hours, with plenty of time between the tests for coffee, conversations, and bathroom breaks.

The reason for this stark time disparity is because there are no patients. In nuclear, we see only data, pictures on screens. There are no human beings, and no human empathy. Empathy can't help you read the path of dye in someone's heart muscle. Instead, we study the paths with wise, experienced readers looking over our shoulders.

The tech administers the test but doesn't read it. He or she is the monitor, making sure the radioactive tracer injection goes in, following each step, and taking care of the patients while they are on the treadmill. After the radioactive tracer is injected, the patients have "resting" images taken of their hearts. Then they exercise while another injection is given, so that a set of "during," or midtest, images is taken. Afterward, a final set of "recovery" images is taken. Nuclear looks at each of these images in order to assess how the heart muscle "uptakes" the radioactive tracer. The manner and the intensity with which the tracer is taken up by different regions of the heart muscle can reveal an area that might not be getting enough blood supply during exertion (stress), which would indicate a possible or developing blockage. Basically, we're looking for traffic jams before an accident occurs.

Although we were given preparatory reading material before starting this rotation, the reality is that we learn by watching the images on the screen and listening to the attending describe what's there. Some attendings are better than others at explaining and passing on their skills. Some are so good at spotting blockages they seem like seers. Reviewing a series of images, the attending will point to an innocuous-looking area and zoom in. "Aha, an occlusion of the right coronary artery." Really? Where? We all nod in agreement, even though we're scrambling to mentally record the image, trying to learn to see as the attending sees.

Every day has a set, calm routine now. I head to the hospital in the afternoon, go into the nuclear lab, and plow through the tests from the previous day. We don't read the results in real time while the test is given. Instead, we log our assessments in a computer report as the test is read, and those assessments are accessible to anyone in the Hopkins network.

Ultimately, there are only two possible errors you can make in nuclear. One is not calling something you should call—an abnormal study you read as normal—in which case, the patient could experience a heart attack because you didn't catch it. The other error is calling something abnormal when there's nothing there. The treating doctor is then obliged to order more tests, medicines, procedures, or even surgery, which may or may not be necessary. I find myself wondering how often invasive, risky, costly procedures are ordered because of a misread stress test. Since few patients complain when their test comes out negative, it's impossible to gauge. Still, there's something about nuclear that plants nagging questions.

But I can't help noticing that the doctors who work in nuclear tend to be calm, relaxed, sane, and older. They go over test after test with remarkable efficiency. A few of them also see patients, which creates a balance of clinical medicine and eyes-on-screen analytics, but most seem content with the steady routine of pure nuclear. It seems that I'm the only one who feels guilty about working shorter days. When I ask another Fellow, "What are we supposed to do with all of our downtime?" he looks at me as if I've lost my mind. "How about sleeping late? How about relaxing? How about nothing?"

I take his advice, and fill my extra time with jogs in the July–August heat and humidity. I catch up on *Meet the Press* and *The New York Times,* and the political figures vying for attention. I plan a trip to see my extended family in Colombia, and I make an effort to see old friends.

I admit to myself, I'm a little bored.

Even though it might be peaceful and relaxing, I realize that hunting for arterial buildup on computer screens is not for me. If anything, this rotation feels too calm, too much like being on the other side of the glass again. It's clear to me, I need to be closer to the front lines, with the patients, despite the sleep deprivation, anxiety, and stress that entails. I need patient interaction. In a more cynical or selfish moment, I recognize that's a costly realization. Too bad I don't like nuclear. It is considered one of the more lucrative areas of cardiology. Every test costs a lot, is reimbursed by an insurance company, and brings revenue to the hospital, the testing service, and the doctor who reads it. But a lucrative career where I never meet a patient, never become one of the doctors who actively work to impact a patient's life . . . that's just not for me.

As the days go by, I find myself itching to get back to bedside medicine. I remind myself that nuclear is a fundamental diagnostic skill. It is supposed to be pure science, and there's a part of me that is drawn to the scientific side of medicine, to the clarity that a diagnosis provides. But the more I study the blots and blobs, the more nuclear feels like a rudimentary version of a videogame, where a series of fuzzy pictures can mean something . . . or nothing. Nuclear perfusion imaging may sound high-powered and impressive, but anything sounds more important if you put the word *nuclear* in front of it. The reality is that the quality of the images is variable at best. It turns out that nuclear is less of a pure science, and more about subjective interpretation.

While we call medicine a science, a good deal of it is the art of reading between the lines, of piecing together clues, of seeing patterns, like squinting at the stars and recognizing dogs and bears and calling them constellations. Even the best doctors, the ones who can practically sense a blockage, rely on intuition and related clues—such as chest and arm pain, shortness of breath, and enzyme elevation—and not just the images. One attending will say, "There's an abnormality," and another will say, "Maybe." They each send their readings to the treating physician, who then has to decide on the next treatment steps.

I would never tell a patient or a relative not to have the

test, or to discount the results. In general, I'd recommend it as useful in the right situation. And I'd pay attention to the results. But to me, nuclear feels like fancy guesswork, an assessment that fails to take in the overall picture. This is my biggest issue with nuclear, and also what makes it the easiest rotation for the doctors: It's a vacuum.

In my final week of nuclear, I come face-to-face with what I find most problematic about these tests. It's not their subjectivity, or the money they bring in, but that their interpretation can be almost totally disconnected from the patient.

It's my last Wednesday on nuclear, which means that today is my day for continuity clinic. Once a week, every Fellow works for a half day at an outpatient clinic connected to the Hopkins system, where we practice cardiology like a fully qualified practitioner. It's a chance to treat people on an ongoing basis and develop a longitudinal, therapeutic relationship with patients over time, all the while improving our skills with pros looking over our shoulders.

I'm assigned to the White Marsh clinic, which presents a stark contrast to the downtown hospital neighborhood. White Marsh is a stereotypical suburb—SUV-driving middle-class families in cul-de-sac developments, ranch homes with granite countertops and big mortgages, upwardly striving people, whose heart issues are perhaps their only commonality with the East Baltimore population.

Two of the patients I see are candidates for nuclear stress tests. The first is Jennifer, a forty-six-year-old woman who seems enviably healthy. She works out five days a week, with no apparent medical problems. Recently, she has developed a pain in the right side of her chest, which comes and goes at random intervals. If she rubs her shoulder, the pain seems to get better. Still, her friend insisted that she see a doctor, so here she is. The attending physician and I take her history and conclude that there's nothing seriously wrong. But, since this assessment does not satisfy Jennifer's anxiety, we order a nuclear stress test to reassure her. Jennifer has the test at the clinic, and it is sent digitally to Hopkins for reading the next day.

Later in the afternoon, I meet Albert, a walking ad for heart disease. During our examination, he rattles off a litany of risk factors: He's fifty-seven years old, obese, has poorly controlled high blood pressure, poorly controlled diabetes, poorly controlled cholesterol, smokes two packs of Marlboro Lights a day (having proudly switched from regulars to lights), and often meets his buddies for lunch at the Burger King near his office. If he walks more than a block or two, he gets a "squeezy pain" on the left side of his chest, which, right out of the textbook, runs down his left shoulder and arm. Amazingly, he isn't too worried, because, "If I sit still and put out my cigarette, it goes away. Then I walk slower." The reason he's here is that his wife nagged him into seeing a heart doctor. In Albert's case, we order a very justified nuclear stress test.

Since I happen to be doing nuclear readings the next day, I actually know something about the people behind the tests. Usually, the test readers know almost nothing about the patient, so this is a fluke. For me, Jennifer isn't just a name on a readout. I know something very important about her: that she's pretty healthy, and there's a low probability of coronary disease. And the test shows nothing. But if I hadn't personally examined her, if I didn't know something about her, then it's possible that she would have been recommended for all kinds of risky, expensive diagnostic procedures to confirm, or reconfirm, that she's a healthy forty-six-year-old woman whose shoulder sometimes hurts.

Now it's Albert's turn. Again, by chance, I know him as a patient, not just as pictures of radioactive dye running through vessels into his muscle cells. I know that he's at the top of the charts for likelihood of coronary diseases. With that knowledge, I study his stress test very carefully for any abnormality. If I didn't know about his deplorable eating habits, his smoking, his "squeezy pain," his method of relieving his arm pain, I would have no understanding of the whole picture. Would I be as suspicious? Would I look as hard?

Tests are tests. They don't have eyes or ears. They don't know background, habits, perspiration, or attitude. They examine openings and flow. They don't talk to people. A test without a conversation, without an understanding of the patient's humanity, seems incomplete to me. Conscientious doctors make the assessments and send patients for tests, but then test readers call an abnormality, or miss it, in a relative vacuum.

As I drive home, I'm relieved to be done with this rotation. Nuclear seems not only a little dull, but frustratingly myopic and inhuman as well. Still, I haven't wasted the last two weeks of my life: Now I know there's no way I'm going to be a nuclear cardiologist.

4

DISTANCE AND PERSPECTIVE

*Sometimes You Have to Get Away
from Medicine to See It Clearly*

I have survived four years of med school, three years of residency, including one year of preparing and applying for fellowship, but after two months of living and breathing cardiology, I realize that I am drained and exhausted. Fellowship is not harder than residency, but it is more intense. Instead of getting a broad overview of a discipline, the point is to immerse ourselves in every detail of cardiology, to understand the minutiae, and then be able to apply it all. This is what it means to be a cardiologist. To be a cardiologist at Johns Hopkins, though, means being steeped in the culture, customs, and language of the hospital. It's easy to forget that there is a world outside of the hospital at all.

I'm hoping that a visit to my family in Medellín, Colombia, will provide the grounding and perspective that I need. It's a trip that I've made several times, usually with my parents and my sister. This time, it's only me. That's okay. I'm glad to be alone, just me and my medical and personal ruminations.

Both of my parents are originally from Medellín; most of our family still lives there, including my grandmothers (both of my grandfathers have passed away). But because I was born and raised in the United States, Colombia was always the place I traveled to, not the place that I came from. When my sister and I were younger, Colombia was the place where we saw our grandparents at Christmas. Some people went to Florida; we went to Colombia. When we got older and heard the news stories of drugs and crime, Colombia seemed like a scary, dangerous place. Now, Medellín is just another big city. It's true that there is rampant hardship in Medellín— too many people trying to live on too little. But the only difference between the drug business in Medellín and in the United States is that in the United States, we can compartmentalize it, or live well in spite of it. I choose to live in Baltimore, a city that a show such as *The Wire* depicts as far more threatening than anything in Medellín. In reality, I have nothing to fear. Visiting Medellín feels like coming full circle, as if I'm leaving my stress and anxiety behind, almost like being a kid again.

Almost. I still have some things on my mind. I'm visiting my roots, and I want to see how my family has contributed to who I am, and what I am trying to be. How did I get here? Who and what made me this way? I've spent so little time here that while my Colombian family are loved ones, they can sometimes feel almost like strangers. I'm trying to connect, to find out what habits or values or DNA they added to the chemical mix that made me into me.

I am staying with my father's mother, the matriarch of the family, who still lives on her own. My father is currently a professor of epidemiology in the United States, but he grew up in Medellín as one of three children. It's home, and while one of his sisters lives in New York, the other lives in the building next door to my grandmother, with her husband and their twenty-three-year-old daughter. Their father—my grandfather—was a successful local attorney in Medellín, who also served for two years as the city's mayor. As a result, the family placed a high value on education. After my father graduated from the university here, he went on to Stanford for his doctorate in mathematics, and from there to Harvard. My father's family may value education in faraway places, but their roots in Medellín are deep.

My maternal grandmother is in an assisted-living facility nearby. My mother is one of ten siblings, and she is the only one no longer in Colombia. Her father was a navy pilot, and he and my grandmother made sure that my mother and her brothers and sisters were well educated—a lesson that my mother clearly took to heart, as she is now a professor of ophthalmology. But what I admire most about my mother is her remarkable inner strength, a quality that I don't yet know if I inherited from her. I want to see for myself whether this resiliency perhaps comes from growing up in Colombia as part of a strong family, able to deal with loss, but possessing an ability to move on.

As I settle into family life here, it seems that the best way to foster a connection is not to ask deep, searching questions but to participate in the international, time-honored tradition of being overfed by your grandmother. Between all these meals with various aunts, uncles, and cousins, I run miles every day in a futile effort to stay even with my calorie intake. I eat and I talk. I run around the courtyard of my grandmother's building and I think.

The house is full of relatives, telling stories, reminiscing, but mostly talking about me and asking questions. The family likes the idea that I'm a doctor. They like the service aspect—that I can help people, and that they will have someone who can listen to them and maybe fix their ailments. But they wonder why becoming a cardiologist takes so many years. As long as they can remember, I've been in school or training of some sort. I often think the same thing. When do you actually get to be what you're training to be one day? When are you done? Yes, when? Although I came here for answers from my relatives, it is their questions that linger.

They're less impressed with credentials, with titles or prestige or names. They're impressed with reality, with whether or not I can help the sick. You're a doctor? That's good. You can make people well? That's good. You went to Johns Hopkins? Or Harvard? Or Stanford? So what? The name of the university doesn't seem to carry the same weight that it does back in the United States. Residency, fellowship, chief of this, or head of that? Titles don't matter. Here in Colombia, they're just the means to the all-important end of healing people.

As the days go by, I find myself venturing outside of my grandmother's neighborhood. I start to explore Medellín itself. I don't always know exactly where I am or where I'm headed, but the more I run, the more I learn my way. Similarly, the more I talk to my relatives, the more I realize that the essence of cardiology is not a competition, a series of victories or losses against heart disease. There's no race.

Their attitude is a dose of humility, and precisely the kind of perspective that I need. Don't take your fancy credentials too seriously. Sick people don't see your grades, or your diploma, or care where you were ranked to match. My relatives say it lovingly, but their message is unmistakable: Get your priorities in order. You have been given special opportunities. Don't waste them. Use them well. Their simple message is like a cold shower. The real challenge is to become a good doctor and learn how to help others. My questions about who I am, my inherited qualities and shared characteristics, appear increasingly irrelevant next to the forthrightness of my Colombian family.

When every day consists of studying charts, diagnosing, prescribing, and staring at EKG lines, it's easy to start thinking that the world revolves around Johns Hopkins and its metrics of success. But the evaluations of the attending doctors, the number of papers published, and even the titles earned are cold and quantitative and often superficial ways to measure progress. Focusing on accolades—even though you work with patients every day—is just another way of placing yourself on the opposite side of the glass.

Thousands of miles away from my fellowship, my relatives assessed me by other gauges—human gauges, values, and worth. After Colombia, I feel cleaner, as if I have washed off some of the superficiality and returned to what mattered, to why I became a cardiologist. On the plane ride back, I think that I've regained the balance I lost. Now the trick will be hanging on to it.

5

FELLOWS' CASE CONFERENCE

My Turn

It's my second day back, my case conference day, a command performance, Johns Hopkins–style, before my peers and my superiors.

In front of me are thirty-five impressive/intimidating doctors in a space that comfortably accommodates fifteen people. This room is normally a combination of meeting room and cafeteria, and it is littered with old paperbacks, empty soda cans, and worn chairs around a battered table. But on Wednesday mornings, it is also the conference room for the Fellows' case conference—and today is my day to present.

The conferences are ongoing teaching sessions through the first two years of the cardiology program in which one Fellow discusses a case with the other Fellows and the cardiology faculty. The conference begins with a twenty- to thirty-minute presentation of the case, including the patient's history, his or her EKG, test results, et cetera. Then come the questions about the patient's history, symptoms, tests—the whole gamut. The attendings ask and field most of the questions. Opinions fly, sometimes flaring into spirited disagreement. The presenter has to steer the conversation toward a consensus on critical factors, course of action, and prognosis. Meanwhile, since the Fellows are there to listen and learn, both the Fellows and the attending staff are scrutinizing the presenter, judging the case selection, the presenter's understanding, and his or her diagnosis. It's billed as a discussion, but you want to look smart, be prepared, and not wing it.

As soon as the case conference dates are set—mine was the second of all the Fellows—you start to consider each patient you meet as a potential candidate for the presentation. Is this case sufficiently interesting? Sufficiently puzzling? Sufficiently multidimensional to generate an hour's worth of discussion? Conferences are clearly the academic, esoteric side of medicine, in contrast to the pragmatic, deliver-basic-care-to-people-who-need-it-now side I'd witnessed during my time in Colombia. Sometimes I have to remind myself that the academic is what leads to better delivery of the pragmatic.

For faculty, attendance is optional, determined by the particular case and its relevance to their subspecialties within cardiology. For Fellows, attendance is "encouraged but not mandatory." My being the second and not the first to present turned out to be significant. At the first case, most of the attendings showed up, but only four Fellows did. Dr. Quincy, who oversees the conferences, wasn't pleased and sent a none-too-subtle email to everyone explaining that when attendance is "encouraged but not mandatory," it means "Be there."

So here we are—room packed.

The case I chose was that of Mr. Zell, a thirty-six-year-old man recently diagnosed with a serious case of acute lymphoblastic leukemia and currently undergoing chemotherapy treatment. At the time, I was on the cardiology consult rotation, and I was asked to see him because a recent CT (computed tomography) scan indicated there was excess fluid around his heart; he was having difficulty breathing, and his heart rate was increasing. We'd first met on a Friday afternoon in a private room at the oncology center. Mr. Zell had his laptop open, his television on, and he was talking on his cell phone via Bluetooth, like someone in a private airline lounge at an airport. This is a surprisingly standard scene in oncology; refusing to give up the routines and diversions of their daily life, whether work or social media, is one way many patients deal with a devastating diagnosis.

The first thing I observed about Mr. Zell was how fast he was breathing. Lying in bed, doing nothing but tapping computer keys, he was huffing and puffing thirty-five times a minute, nearly double the normal respiratory rate. There were several possible reasons for his breathing difficulties: Does he have pneumonia? Does he have a blood clot in his lungs (a pulmonary embolism)? Does he have congestive heart failure? Does he have excess fluid in the sac that surrounds his heart? Finding the primary culprit was critical: Excess fluid around the heart can be extremely dangerous because it creates pressure on the heart. Enough fluid and the heart chambers can collapse, like what divers' lungs face in deep, pressurized water. With this in mind, I had one of the echo techs set Mr. Zell up for an echocardiogram, the ultrasound procedure that would reveal whether the fluid was compressing the heart, and force us toward a decision point: Should we go in with a needle and take the fluid out? And if so, should we do it immediately or should we wait? If the patient's heart rate or blood pressure drops precipitously, or if the patient is unstable or "coding," the answer is clearly "immediately." But when the patient's condition is less obviously dire, there is a chance that the problem might stabilize, or even slowly improve on its own. If there's any reasonable chance that things will get better without intervention, it's preferable to sidestep the risk of an invasive procedure, especially in a patient whose immune system and blood cell counts have been weakened by chemotherapy. With his body's defenses in a compromised state, Mr. Zell would be at higher risk of developing an infection from any invasive procedure. But waiting can be risky, since waiting itself can eventually precipitate an emergency, and any procedure that has the word *emergency* as a modifier is inherently more risky.

By Friday evening, the tech has performed the ultrasound. Mr. Zell's heart already shows signs of early collapse in the right-sided heart chambers, the right atrium and right ventricle. It's not an official emergency yet, but I don't see the situation getting better. The problem appears to be chemo-related, but Mr. Zell needs the chemotherapy for the cancer. I write up my impressions and present them to Dr. George, and he agrees. Sooner or later, Mr. Zell needs to have this

fluid drained, and we don't want to wait until he "crumps"—
medical slang for "fail fast."

Dr. George and I go to see Mr. Zell, now with his wife at
his bedside. There seems to be some sort of traditional machismo in play, as Mr. Zell is still insisting that he's "fine"
despite his constant gasping and panting. We explain to him
that his condition is not life-threatening at this moment but
that it could be soon. "The chemotherapy, which you have to
have for your cancer, is the most likely cause of the fluid ac-
cumulation around your heart. It won't get better on its own.
We think it's time to consider having the fluid drained." We
carefully explain the procedure—pericardiocentesis—which
involves inserting a long needle through the chest wall, into
the pericardium, or sac that surrounds the heart muscle, and
then withdrawing fluid from the pericardial sac until the
pressure is relieved. Mr. Zell listens calmly, as if we were suggesting it might be time to get a haircut.

After we finish, he says, "I'll wait." We're stunned. Dr.
George says, "Our recommendation is to do it today, but we
can watch you closely to try to avoid this becoming an emergency." Mr. Zell nods and we exit.

But his wife follows us out of the room, saying, "Is it dangerous?" Is she asking whether his condition is dangerous or
whether the procedure is? Or both? If she's like most people,
Mrs. Zell heard "long needle," "through the chest wall," "into
the heart muscle"—and it sounded dangerous. In fact, it's
not a needle into the heart; the interventional cardiology
team uses ultrasound and X-ray guidance to place the needle into the sac around the heart, an important distinction
in terms of potential harm. The procedure carries risk, but
it's often done without incident in the cath lab, where the

team watches every second of the needle's insertion on a monitor to make sure that the needle's path steers clear of the heart itself. But in an emergency, the pericardiocentesis can be done at the patient's bedside, and we have to go in "anatomically"—which means that the team is aiming for the fluid collection without the video assistance of ultrasound or X rays. Mr. Zell's decision to delay potentially makes his situation more dangerous.

Saturday passes. Before I go home, I find the intern on call and tell him to check on Mr. Zell throughout the night and alert me if anything occurs. The intern's reaction is to wonder why anyone of sound thinking would wait. I can't help but agree—I'm fully prepared to get a 2:00 a.m. page that reads, "Mr. Zell is crumping."

But when I return to the hospital on Sunday, it seems that Mr. Zell has changed his mind and is ready to have the procedure. Maybe he saw the light. Maybe his wife convinced him. Maybe he felt worse. Or maybe being asked "Are you okay?" every few minutes by a nervous intern on call rattled him. Nothing does more to convince you that you're not okay than someone constantly asking if you are.

I show both the "before" and "after" echocardiograms at the case conference. I want my audience's opinions as to whether Mr. Zell's heart chambers were in partial (i.e., early) collapse or full (i.e., more advanced) collapse. Neither answer is great, but one is definitely worse. Then, depending on their conclusions, what would they have done? Would they have pushed as hard or harder to tap him earlier? Would they have labeled it an emergency? Was the fluid around the heart the direct result of the chemo? Would they have presented the situation differently to Mr. and Mrs. Zell?

As I lay out the facts of the case, I am nervously trying to gauge the reaction of my audience. Basically, there are two nightmare scenarios for a case conference: Nightmare A is when you present to total silence, not because you've stunned the listeners with your brilliance but because your case is so obvious that there's nothing to discuss. In that nightmare, one of the attendings says, "Simple, straightforward, and no reason to be here at this early hour." Nightmare B also ends in silence, but this time it's because your case is a statistical outlier, highly unlikely to recur, and therefore of little or no value. In that version, one of the attendings says, "Fascinating. Ellis–van Creveld syndrome, traced to a rare autosomal recessive trait, found in Amish people, resulting in atrial septal defects, sometimes manifesting in extra digits and dwarfism. That should be very helpful should a case come along again in this century."

I open the discussion by fielding questions from some of the Fellows, and then the faculty members weigh in. After scrutinizing the films, some faculty members see this as an open-and-shut case—the procedure should have been done immediately. Others think you could make a case, albeit a thin one, for waiting. The nuances of reading the films have proved, once again, that these tests are not yes/no data points but rather pictures subject to interpretation. What is "collapsed" to one set of eyes is "almost collapsed" to another. What is "a lot of fluid" to one expert is "too much fluid" to another. What constitutes an emergency is sometimes a matter of opinion. It is our job to make the subjective as objective as possible, to try to turn art into science—but even a roomful of experts cannot always reach a consensus.

Still, there is widespread agreement that we gave the patient and his wife an accurate picture of the situation and, if anything, would have been justified in being more dramatic. Success: The attendings and the Fellows believe that the case was handled appropriately. One attending even cracks that the patient's denial reminds him of the scene in *Monty Python and the Holy Grail* where the Black Knight has limb after limb hacked off by King Arthur in a duel. Even when the knight is nothing but a head and a torso on the ground, he still insists, "It's just a flesh wound!"

We all laugh, and the group files out. Good questions. Good answers. No nightmare scenarios. I survived. Then I remember Colombia and the conversations I had with myself on priorities and realities. In the real world, no one cares about your who's-smarter-than-who meetings or fancy credentials or elite hospitals, only about being sick and finding someone to help you get better. Yes, I made it through Fellows' case conference, but what about Mr. Zell, his cancer, and the fluid around his heart? Whose outcome is important here? A Fellow's or the patient's? How do I keep my perspective as I continue through more rotations, more training, and ultimately more years of practice?

6

ROTATION: PREVENTIVE CARDIOLOGY, PART I

Patient, Heal Thyself

The day after the case conference, I drive into the main hospital parking lot to begin the initial two-week segment of a four-week rotation in preventive cardiology. (I'll do the second part of it in a few months.) It's a clinical rotation, which means that we see patients all day, every day at Hopkins's Center for the Prevention of Heart Disease.

And it's intense. Not in the sense of endless days, sleepless nights, and dramatic paddles-to-the-chest resuscitation, but because of the single-minded determination to reform and alter a patient's lifestyle, to rewire human behavior from a live-for-today to a live-to-see-tomorrow attitude. On top of that, the center itself is so well respected that it is almost synonymous with the practice of preventive cardiology as a whole. It's a team of true believers whose members live, breathe, and eat (in moderation, of course) what they do.

Their leader is Dr. Franklin, a lanky and lean, six foot four sixty-year-old who looks more like a small forward for a Division III college basketball team than the embodiment of preventive heart care at Hopkins. I've heard that Dr. Franklin went to medical school with the idea of becoming a sports team physician or Olympic training doctor but that his interests in the heart evolved when he came to Hopkins for his cardiology fellowship. He helped to establish the center, and preventive has been his passion ever since.

At first glance, Dr. Franklin's office looks like a heart condition hall of fame. The walls are adorned with pictures of him next to somebody famous—a professional athlete, a coach, a team owner, a politician, a writer, an executive. It seems that even world-renowned specialists such as Dr. Franklin can have a weakness for stars. But Dr. Franklin speaks so enthusiastically about the work he does that it becomes clear that these pictures serve an ulterior purpose. He's dedicated, almost religiously, to preventive cardiology. He'll do anything to advance the cause and fortify the temple, the Center for the Prevention of Heart Disease. That takes money. And stars—business, Hollywood, sports, political—have access to money, whether it's through their own deep pockets or through their affiliations with foundations, important donors, or sources of government funding.

The center also needs young cardiologists. Not very subtly, Dr. Franklin wants to get me, and as many of the other Fellows as possible, interested in a career in preventive. He says, "The point of these two weeks is to teach you as much about prevention as possible, and have you see the patients," then hands me a stack of articles on the latest prevention guidelines and adds, "When you get a chance, read these over and let me know what you think. There may be some ways we can improve upon these published guidelines." I can't tell whether he seriously believes that I, a Fellow in training, can actually improve the guidelines or he's trying to woo me into his field through challenge and flattery. In either case, he leaves me feeling that the future of the guidelines rests on my shoulders ... which makes me want to perform at my best, so his methods work.

For the next two weeks, my role is to be Dr. Franklin's advance man at the clinic: I'm him until he gets there. As the head of preventive cardiology, Dr. Franklin sees the patients with significant risk factors—very high cholesterol, very high blood pressure, pronounced family history of heart disease, major heart events—and/or the famous and powerful people who are concerned they might develop a serious heart problem.

For the first half hour, I see the patients, take their history, do the preliminary examination, and look at their charts, so that when Dr. Franklin walks in, I have a summary ready: "Mr. McDonnell is back for his regular yearly visit, and here are the issues. . . ." Normally, the next step is for Dr. Franklin to ask his own questions and draw his own conclusions— but what he does first is formally introduce me to each of his patients as well. "Mr. McDonnell, Dr. Muñoz is one of our finest cardiology Fellows, a graduate of Johns Hopkins Med School and residency, whom we're honored to have in our program. Dr. Muñoz is destined to be one of the stars of the field." This introduction may sound impressive, but the reality is that it's better than the alternative: "This is Dr. Muñoz. He's just learning to be a cardiologist."

Once the flattery is over, Dr. Franklin zeroes in on key

areas, based on his experience and instinct: It could be the patient's cholesterol, blood pressure, most recent EKG, or even how the patient reports feeling. With every patient, we ask the same questions—habits, meals, snacking, drinking, work patterns, stress levels, family history, prior treatment. And with every one, Dr. Franklin uses the patient's answers to piece together what appears to be a custom-tailored routine that he is careful to call "our" plan: "Dan and I feel that the best course would be . . . ," or "I concur with Dr. Muñoz's recommendation for a test of . . ." In reality, the conclusions are his, but his implication that I've been an integral part of generating the recs is part of his teaching and subtle recruiting method. He is constantly enlisting those around him—Fellows into his preventive enterprise, patients into adopting better approaches to their health. It's strong-arming with a smile, rather than through fear or intimidation.

Nearly every patient's plan follows an ordered mnemonic device known as A-B-C-D-E. A is aspirin; B is blood pressure control or beta-blockers; C is cholesterol; D is diet; E is exercise. Dr. Franklin hits every one, in order, with every patient, and he does it in a conversation, connected by clues the patient gives him.

In most cases, the people who visit the center are still relatively healthy. A forty-year-old man comes in, panicking because his dad died of a heart attack at age forty and he now thinks his own arteries might be closing. A woman comes in with dangerously high cholesterol, even though she hasn't eaten fatty food in two years—just a case of bad genetics. Another guy is flirting with disaster because he smokes, is gaining weight, can't walk a block without panting, and wakes up every third night with chest pains. Here's a diet.

Here's a calorie count. Here's a portion-control guide. Here's an exercise regime. Here's your target weight. Make an appointment for six months from now. It could easily get mundane.

But even when the patient gets the standard A-B-C-D-E review, Dr. Franklin makes the effort to create a personal connection: "Middle-aged paunch? We all get it." "You play golf? Me too. I never take a cart. Walking relaxes me, and you get three miles of exercise." He will tell patients to lose five pounds instead of twenty-five because twenty-five is discouraging, but an initial five is doable. His method is so smooth and natural that it is almost an art form. He says, "Switch to Miller Lite," even though he means, "Stop drinking beer." But Dr. Franklin wants allies, not enemies—he understands how people work and think. It's my job to learn by observation, and I'm truly struck by Dr. Franklin's deftness in plying his craft, how attuned he is to each patient's personality, cooperation, or level of resistance. He seems to have mastered the notion that practicing medicine is more than just a series of tests and cases; he grasps that being a doctor is more than just the procedures that save lives, but also involves the lives that the patients lead. Again, this brings to mind my recent thoughts on the basic human need for practical, effective, realistic doctors. And it drives home to me that this is the kind of responsiveness and empathy I want to master.

Dr. Franklin's ability to listen and connect to his patients also means that they are often extremely well informed. They know their own conditions and take an interest in the preventive practices that can change their fates. They can rattle off their family histories, their parents' cholesterol levels, as well as their own levels, exercise routines, and weight goals. Sometimes, they even speak the language of heart disease, using words like *triglycerides* and *stent* and *bypass* as easily as other people spout sports jargon. They become proactive authorities on their own health—and all because Dr. Franklin gets through to them.

It helps that Dr. Franklin practices what he preaches. He wears a fitness tracker at all times and is a "walking" ad for it, directing patients to a website that sells them. Every day he measures how many steps he takes, with his personal goal of ten thousand steps, or five miles, in mind. At the end of the day, if he comes up short, he takes the stairs in the parking garage. If he's still short, he walks around his neighborhood with his wife. On weekends he still plays basketball and lacrosse, and boasts a single-digit handicap in golf. He coaches neighborhood kids' sports teams as well. He eats right. The message to patients is clear: If I can do this, so can you. By the time we finish an exam, the patients always seem rededicated to losing another five pounds, walking farther, doing more push-ups, or lowering their stress. And I'm recharged to go to the next exam room.

During the rotation, I also work with the other doctors on Dr. Franklin's team, each of whom specializes in a specific aspect of prevention. One is the world's expert on lipids and cholesterol, and sees only patients who have horrifically high cholesterol. Like Dr. Franklin, he combs through the clues of each patient's lifestyle, looking for ways to modify his or her behavior, and prescribe the right combination of drugs to stave off deadly LDL (low-density lipoprotein) advancement.

Two days later, I follow the team's ace diabetes doctor.

Our first patient, Adele, is forty-five years old, five foot two, and weighs 212 pounds. She has two daughters: a sixteen-year-old who is the same height and weight as her mother, and an eight-year-old who already weighs more than 100 pounds. Since diabetes is a significant risk factor for coronary disease, controlling it helps prevent heart trouble. But the converse is also true: If the patient can't control his or her diabetes, the probability of coronary disease skyrockets.

Adele is on cholesterol medication and following a diet that she is struggling to maintain. She and her daughters live on her welfare check, and for better or worse, it goes pretty far at the neighborhood fast-food joints. Since she started coming to the clinic six months ago, she's lost fifteen pounds, but her weight loss has plateaued since her last visit three months ago. The doctor says, "You've made some progress. Keep it up. What did you eat this week?" She tells him, and he winces. He encourages her to cut back on fried foods, to go to KFC no more than twice a week. Adele promises to try. Her younger daughter, hearing only "KFC" in an otherwise dull conversation, asks, "Can we go on the way home?"

This doctor, dealing with the consequences of diabetes daily, preaches some version of this to a patient population that grows every year, figuratively and literally. Obesity is becoming commonplace in America, and diabetes, unfortunately, often coincides with obesity. According to the Centers for Disease Control, from the late 1990s to 2014, the incidence of diabetes in the United States more than doubled. Type 2, formerly known as adult diabetes, is now rampant in a substantial portion of adolescents and young adults. The size of the problem and of the patients is not a fluke; it's driven by business—supersized, sweetened, salted, corn oil–

injected, drive-through, fast and cheap food—and exacerbated by a lack of physical activity.

That night, I drive out of the clinic parking lot, and in the space of ten blocks I count six high-cholesterol chains: KFC, Applebee's, Wendy's, Burger King, Pizza Hut, and Bob Evans. Suddenly, I have a craving for a plate of wings or nachos. But after a day of working alongside Dr. Franklin and his team, observing the effects of fast food and sedentary lifestyles, I change my mind and opt for a run and a salad. Still, my moment of weakness highlights what is most difficult and frustrating about preventive cardiology. We know a lot about diabetes, what doctors can do, what patients should do. But preventive cardiology requires the patient's initiative, and its success relies on his or her ability to master every single moment of weakness, to consciously choose salads and push-ups over cookies and sleeping in. Preventive isn't just fighting heart disease; it's also an uphill battle against human nature.

Even the most successful, educated, and privileged people can fall into, and become comfortable with, their bad habits. Plenty of Dr. Franklin's celebrity patients—the business tycoons, movie moguls, pro athletes, media stars, Washington politicos, and Wall Street executives—ignore his wisdom. They may try to follow their plan, but they struggle exactly the way Adele and her daughters do. And some of them just want medicine to "fix" the problem.

In the middle of my second week, we see a certified hotshot who has been referred to us by his internist. The patient, Mr. Gardner, was an Ivy League undergrad who went to an Ivy League law school and is now an attorney at a prestigious firm for high-profile clients. He wears an expensive suit and is articulate and funny—not arrogant, totally likable. Once a track athlete, he still looks fit enough to run the hundred-yard dash. But these days he can't run a hundred feet without getting winded. His cholesterol levels are off the charts, with high blood pressure to match, unlucky genes that he shares with his father and his older brother. In fact, his family is the reason he's here: Mr. Gardner is devoted to his wife and two kids, and his wife made a point of bugging him until he agreed to come to the center.

In the course of our conversation, it quickly becomes clear that the patient is a denier. Dr. Franklin's questions and Mr. Gardner's answers are revealing. He tells us how good he feels, and how tough he is. He apologizes for wasting our time, and says he shouldn't be here, that he came only to mollify his wife. Even as he recounts the story of his father's two massive coronaries—complete with ambulance, EMTs pounding on his father's chest, and a subsequent bypass operation—he jokes that he's too young to worry, and that his high cholesterol and blood pressure are just by-products of representing fat cats in court and racking up billable hours. Even the fact that his older brother is going through the same situation—same genetics, same symptoms—doesn't seem to alarm him. Instead, he cracks a joke: "My brother is four years older, and he never could catch me on the lacrosse field."

Dr. Franklin recognizes the challenge of getting through to Mr. Gardner. Before laying out the plan for prevention, Dr. Franklin takes an interesting tack. "Mr. Gardner, you're an active, successful guy. That's great. But I worry, not about how you feel now, but about the risk of a heart attack or a stroke. And I want to do everything we can to avoid either of those two scenarios. It's in our power to do so, but only if you acknowledge the importance of prevention and the serious consequences of failing to engage in it. A heart attack would sideline you from many of the things you enjoy doing. Your family history suggests you're at risk. We can't control your genes, so let's focus on the things we *can* control."

Mr. Gardner is, for the first time, quiet and appears to be listening.

Dr. Franklin then lays out a plan: diet, exercise, medication, and regular monitoring. This is serious treatment for a serious problem. For a moment, it looks as if the patient gets it. But then he jokes, "I should pass this advice on to my brother and bill him for it." Mr. Gardner knows what to do, and he has the means and the support system to do it. But will he start the regimen to change his life? Or will he put it off "until it's really a problem," when he's on a gurney with EMTs hovering over him? This is my biggest issue with preventive medicine: Because it aims to be routinely proactive, it is far too easy for patients from all walks of life to ignore.

No matter how often he repeats the same conversations, it's clear that Dr. Franklin isn't bored by this routine. Preventive cardiology is the most important thing in the world to him, and after spending two weeks by his side, I find that some of his enthusiasm has rubbed off on me. Though it delivers essentially the same lessons to twenty different people a day, preventive is all about the ripple effect. If more doctors help more patients change their behavior, then little by little, these incremental changes can accomplish a lot. Twenty patients a day, year in and year out, and all for the hope that one day, you will read that the average person is living to be eighty-five instead of eighty-two. This is Dr. Franklin's purpose in life. It's why he writes books and makes speeches, raises money, wants to win over Fellows, and tries to get every patient to make at least some progress. But is it for me?

Dr. Franklin helps people every single day, and he is both a compassionate cardiologist and a practitioner of such skill that he makes it look effortless. But gross tracking of populations, trends, and life expectancy means that it is hard to ascribe success to any single treatment or factor. And he's battling not a disease, but risk: an unpredictable, resilient enemy that constantly fights back, and will surge forward in one area even when he defeats it in another. In an instant, it can attack and sabotage years of good effort. By definition, you can only reduce risk but not fully eliminate it. You can't win. Have you then failed? Have you lost a life? Or is success simply holding off the inevitable for as long as possible?

In medicine, heroic procedures that defy death for the moment gain more attention than steady, behavior-changing routines. A clinical cardiologist tests for and diagnoses heart disease in order to prescribe medication that will relieve debilitating symptoms. In the process, she may slow the disease and save a life. An interventional cardiologist puts in a stent and opens an artery, thereby perhaps staving off a coronary incident. Again, he may save a life. Practicing preventive medicine is the opposite of the dramatic interventions that you see on television. Instead, the goal is to keep these scenes from ever happening and stall death for years, even decades. But how do preventive cardiologists know when they've made a difference?

I've finished my third rotation, but I am still unsure whether preventive is for me. Could I see the same case with a different name over and over again without getting bored? Would I get frustrated wondering whether each patient was hearing my exhortations but choosing to ignore them? Would the big-picture successes be enough reward for the daily battles against beer and nachos?

7

ROTATION: HEART FAILURE AND HEART TRANSPLANTATION, PART I

Who Gets a Heart, Who Doesn't

Heart failure and heart transplantation. The title alone sounds like the stuff of action movies. The hero's heart stops. He's put on life support. A clock ticks as the camera cuts to hotshot doctors ducking under the blades of a helicopter, racing to the gory accident scene. A beating heart is harvested from a clinically dead donor, put "on ice" in an Igloo cooler, and handed off to surgeons who place the heart in the patient. The music swells as the surgeons disconnect the hero from life support, and . . . the heart beats! Fade to black.

That scenario does happen, but not quite like that. While it is true that the harvesting process must be done quickly to keep the donor heart healthy, the reality is more tedious and bureaucratic. There must be documented donor approval for removal, plus lab tests to verify the condition of the heart and the blood type. Nor is it done by cardiovascular disease

Fellows such as me. Heart transplants are performed by cardiovascular surgeons, and the procedures are almost always meticulously planned, carefully executed, with no Hollywood special effects or music.

As cardiologists, not cardiac surgeons, we deal with the patient's heart failure while he or she waits for a transplant. It is our job to keep the patient as healthy as we can, essentially acting as a pit crew for the body. If the transplant is a success, we manage the patient after surgery, keeping him or her alive and well. Our part can be exhilarating—definitely life or death—but no one makes movies about us.

For me, this four-week rotation is a 180-degree transition from trying to head off heart disease in preventive cardiology to trying to reverse heart disease that is already running rampant. Heart failure is not the same as a heart attack. It is a physical state of disease in which the heart muscle is literally failing or dying. Heart failure can be caused by reduced blood supply to the heart muscle, a buildup of blockages in blood flow through the arteries, high blood pressure, deterioration of one or more of the heart valves, or failure of the heart muscle itself. It can be treated with medication and lifestyle changes, and sometimes with surgical intervention such as stent implantation and advanced heart-pump placement. When all else fails, it can mean a heart transplant. In essence, the rotation boils down to one thing: The patients' hearts are unable to keep their bodies adequately perfused with the nutrients they need to stay alive.

I picture what I'll face: patients far sicker than any I saw as a med student or resident, patients whose congestive heart failure no longer responds to medication and who are now flirting with death. Either they are suffering from an acute issue that we're trying to fix without recourse to a heart transplant, they're vying or waiting for a transplant, or they've already had a transplant but have developed a complication.

Given the gravity of what we're about to do, I was prepared for a structured indoctrination: "Today you are about to embark on the most perilous endeavor in your cardiovascular education. . . ." But there is no indoctrination. Instead, I walk into the hospital at 7:30 a.m., just like every other day in fellowship. Still, I want my own take on who's who and what they have before making rounds with the attending. I head up to the CICU (cardiac intensive care unit) and meet patient after patient: "Good morning, Mrs. Carson, I'm Dr. Muñoz. No, Dr. Smith [the last Fellow] is no longer on this rotation. You've been in the CICU since [check date] with severe breathing problems and [check notes for details] . . ." I don't have to do this, and I'm not doing it to earn points. I am doing it because it's my nature to be neurotic and detail-oriented—and often, the extra time spent turns out to be justified.

Another reason for this extra preparation is that this rotation is a crash course in what, until now, we have studied only in an academic setting—the effects of chronic immunosuppression. The immune system is supposed to keep you alive by detecting anything alien in your body—pollen, smog, bacteria, viruses, infection, disease, parasites, poison, or an organ that doesn't belong to you—and rejecting it. If we can suppress the immune system with medication, we can fool the body into accepting an alien liver, kidney, or heart, but, in the process, we leave the body vulnerable to every other kind of attack. Without the normal defenses, something as minor as a sniffle in an elevator or germs from a grandchild can turn into a cold. That cold can become a lung infection, which creates respiratory failure, which builds up fluid that strains the new heart and puts the patient in imminent danger. And it happens every day in hospitals across the country. Pneumonia, flu, diarrhea, or that sniffle can ultimately kill a person whose immune system is down. And hospitals are full of sick people. So even when immunosuppressed patients are shielded from the outside world, their proximity to other patients can endanger them.

Fortunately, there's a cadre of talented doctors who have devoted their lives to studying how to dial the immune system up or down for the maximum effect, to trick the body while putting the patient at minimum risk. After the transplanted organ gets past the new host body's initial resistance, and if it is fully accepted into the body, the immunosuppressants are gradually, but never totally, dialed down, which allows the patient's body to build up resistance to infection and disease. In the meantime, the patient is kept in as safe an environment as possible. But reality rarely plays by the book. The dialing up and down of the immune system seems as much guesswork as science. As a result, chronic immunosuppression is a constant, precarious balancing act between organ rejection and disease invasion.

The attending is Dr. James, whose list of degrees, credentials, and papers makes him a heavy hitter even by Hopkins's standards. Once a West Coast surfer type, he is a longtime Hopkins veteran, with rimless glasses, longish gray hair, and no tie. Above all, he is unflappable. As we make rounds, it becomes clear that Dr. James can get a little bored with the simple cases and often gravitates toward the more exotic. If a patient's heart failure is a result of not taking prescribed medications, Dr. James gives a one-line summary and moves on. But if the case is more challenging, he becomes more thoughtful, takes a longer look at the chart, asks more questions, and turns to me for my thoughts. His training approach is executive style: I trust you. Give me the details that matter. What do you think we should do?

The patients in the CICU range from the very sick but not in imminent danger, to the very sick and in danger but temporarily fixable, to the gravely sick who need a heart soon, to those too sick to get a heart, plus several who change overnight from one category to another. This means constantly weighing two possible conclusions: Is the patient progressing enough to eventually go home, or, if not, could he or she be a candidate for more advanced therapies, such as a transplant? The reality is that it's rare for a patient to check in to the CICU, immediately get placed on a transplant list, and then get whisked away to the OR (operating room). This happens only when the patient's decline is so precipitous that he or she cannot go home but still meets the criteria for a transplant, if a compatible heart can be found fast. More often, patients are put on the transplant list and then go home to wait . . . and hope they live long enough for the call: "Come in. Your new heart is here." A patient could spend months, even years, on the list, with deteriorating odds; a good candidate at the beginning can sometimes become a weak candidate later.

A transplant is not just another operation. It means mobilizing vast resources, people, talents, rooms, equipment, commitments, and finances. The hospital wants all operations to be equally successful, but some operations—

transplants—are more equal than others. Though there are approximately three thousand patients on the national heart transplant wait list each year, only about two thousand hearts become available annually, most often from victims of injuries that have left the heart unscathed. As a result, the wait time on the list varies greatly, from fifty days to well over five hundred. It's brutal but simple math. Hundreds of candidates each year never receive a heart.

But sizing up patients for transplants is about more than just the obvious factors, such as blood type. Having someone else's heart placed inside of you is a major undertaking for both your body and your mind. The heart, unlike almost any other organ, carries symbolic overtones that are impossible to ignore: Your heart is your essence, your emotional center. Even the smallest details, both objective and subjective—patient history, illnesses, genetics, habits, foibles, fears—may affect the fate of a transplant. How will you react to having someone else's essence in you? Will you think or act differently? Are you not only physically but psychologically prepared for a second chance, a new life? On a very practical level, will you take the immunosuppressant medications that will fend off organ rejection and thus keep you alive? The surgery is physically brutal and exhausting; the recovery, long and draining. If the mind cannot help the body, the ordeal will be all but impossible. It's up to the mind not only to make the emotional adjustment but to then be the conscience that ensures the body takes its anti-rejection medicines and shows up at appointments and doesn't play Russian roulette with its new organ. Even after a patient receives a transplant, it is still our responsibility to do the post-transplant biopsies to make sure that the heart tissue remains healthy. This means spending time in the cath lab, looking for evidence of rejection on a cellular level. The resounding lesson of heart failure and heart transplantation is that every single detail, from the patients' mood to their cell tissue, matters.

Still, the extraordinary becomes the ordinary fast. What scares the hell out of you on Monday is a day's work by Wednesday. It's not that we take things for granted; we just become less intimidated and more conditioned about what to expect. Patient after patient comes in with congestive heart failure, and we do temporary fixes—diet adjustments such as salt reduction, diuretics to get rid of fluid buildup, blood pressure medications, ACE inhibitors (which lower arteriolar, or small artery, resistance), beta-blockers to relax the heart and fend off arrhythmias.

We see a youngish grandfather who has come in for his routine "oil change": His fluid retention needs to be flushed out with IV medication. His blood pressure is up; he's short of breath and needs rest. We decide to monitor him until he's out of the danger zone, and with luck, we'll be able to send him home. Another patient has been referred to us by a semirural hospital in the northern suburbs. The doctors there saw a weak heart and some kidney failure—beyond what they felt they could handle—and sent him to us. Is he a candidate for a transplant? We'll see.

Deciding whether a patient is a candidate for a heart transplant is a very human decision on one level, but a very cold and calculated one on another. If the key metrics—age, weight, organ function, test scores, levels, and readings—don't make sense, you cannot responsibly go forward. There just aren't enough donor hearts, and adding someone to the list when the key metrics aren't auspicious means that another candidate might never get the transplant that he or she needs, and possibly deserves, more. One example of this is Mrs. Rabinovich, an overweight, mildly diabetic fifty-six-year-old. She is a former weekend jock and a breast cancer survivor, but she has also had numerous myocardial infarctions and is now in severe congestive heart failure. Is she a candidate? As a cancer survivor, she is resilient and there is a chance that she would be able to survive, and thrive, with a new heart. Although she is stable for the moment, the reality is she's still facing a limited, sedentary life, breathing hard just walking across the room. On the other hand, neither her diabetes nor her weight (things within her control) are well-managed, perhaps signaling that she is not yet ready to take the necessary responsibility for a new organ. As often is the case, it's a judgment call.

The Friday of my first week, we see Mr. Bundy, a returning patient who is gaining weight and whose fondness for over-indulgence is loading his body with salt, resulting in fluid retention. This kind of case may bore Dr. James, but since I'm new to the field, it interests me. Mr. Bundy is breathing hard, almost gasping for air when I ask him to stand up at the side of his bed. His blood pressure is unacceptably high, and he's scared. I can't help but wonder what made him think he could go beer for beer with his nephews. Did it slip his mind that he has a bad heart? Judging from his wife's glares, they've already had this conversation. He stares at the floor and says, "Can you hook me up to that IV medicine, doctor, and get this fluid out of me? Usually, eighty milligrams of IV Lasix works for me. . . ." Our goal is to stabilize him, to see if he takes a turn for the better (unlikely) or for the worse (more likely). In the meantime, he remains a viable candidate for a heart transplant. Over the next twenty-four hours, Mr. Bundy responds to the medication and his body rallies. Three days later, we are able to send him home.

Another case is that of Ms. Francis. In her midforties, she is in excellent physical shape and seems too young, too lean, and too healthy to be in a cardiac care unit. A weekend athlete and the full-time CFO of a construction company, she's managed to achieve gender equality in a male-dominated field: an impressive testament to her will and force of character. Ms. Francis also has bad genes on both sides of her family: Her mother died young, her father has severe coronary artery disease, both sets of grandparents had heart issues, and she survived a heart attack less than a year ago. Last week she had fevers and cold symptoms. She got steadily worse, developing a case of viral myocarditis, an inflammation of the heart muscle that can result in heart muscle function deteriorating rapidly, sometimes within days, and was now at death's door in the cardiac intensive care unit. Given her deterioration, Ms. Francis undergoes an expedited evaluation. Dr. James and our team review and rereview her chart, her vitals, and most important, the human factor, Ms. Francis herself. I weigh in. Together we perform our best assessment of her outcome. Dr. James makes the call. She will be recommended to go on the heart transplant list.

Doctors want to make rational, measured decisions, but most cases are not as purely rational and measured as we'd like. Some conditions change over time, with circumstances, with developments in science. In 1985, patients with HIV never received organ transplants. At the time, there was no long-term treatment for HIV; the prevailing wisdom was that if you were going to die of that disease, that new heart would be of more use to someone else. Now that there are treatments that can keep HIV patients healthy, they're more often considered for certain organ transplants. But the truth is, we're making not just scientific, but moral and ethical judgments. Although there are guidelines, processes, and metrics that try to make these decisions as clear-cut as possible, the fact is that our profession grants us the power of life and death over fellow human beings.

One night, after a long day on the rotation, I can't sleep as I try to unwind this mental dilemma. Why are we allowed to make these calls over people's fates? Who are we to decide? It's fair. It's not fair. Someone has to do it. No one should do it. As doctors, we are better qualified than most because we know the diseases and the risk factors involved. But what about the intangibles—the value of one person's life over another's? We have no way of knowing which person might do more for humanity or who might be a better father, mother, friend, or colleague. We aren't philosophers or priests or gurus. Maybe we shouldn't do transplants at all. But then more people would die. I look at the clock and realize that it's 4:40 a.m. In two hours, I'll go back to work, where these questions won't be rhetorical, and where these decisions will still have to be made.

The next day, Dr. James and I meet Malcolm. He's not the kind of case you see often, which means that he has Dr. James's full attention. Malcolm is six foot four, a muscular former college wrestler, now mechanic, who had just turned thirty-three. My initial impression was that Malcolm looked exactly the way you'd expect a former wrestler to look. Nothing about him denoted frailty . . . until he needed to string together more than a few words, and then he had to work to catch his breath. And while most athletes tend to have low resting heart rates, in the range of 60 to 75 beats per minute, Malcolm's resting heart rate was around 135. Even though he was in bed, hooked up to IVs and monitors, his heart rate was closer to what it would have been during his wrestling matches in college. He hadn't made bad lifestyle decisions, had no bad habits, or even apparently bad genes. Although he hadn't started to feel "different" until recently, he had told himself that his shortness of breath and inexplicable weight gain were just part of getting older, middle age coming on. But one day, he noticed that his legs were swollen as well, and had decided to see a doctor.

At first, he'd been prescribed antibiotics for pneumonia. When he didn't get better, his doctors tried treatments for other illnesses. But Malcolm was still tired, still out of breath, and his legs were still swelling. And then he had a heart attack—and not the mild, cheeseburgers-and-fries kind, but one caused by a thrombus, a painful, life-threatening blood clot in one of his arteries. In the cath lab, they located and sucked out the thrombus, and put in a stent to keep the artery open. But despite the evidence of Malcolm's chest pain, his EKG, and his enzyme levels, it wasn't a typical heart attack: It was the result of underlying heart failure.

A patient suffers a heart attack when a blood vessel or artery is blocked. Heart failure occurs when the heart itself is the issue—and Malcolm's heart was huge. It was dilated and functioning at a barely adequate level. A healthy heart has an ejection fraction of 60 to 65 percent, which means that of the possible 100 percent of the blood that the left ventricle ejects with each heartbeat, about two-thirds of it flows out into the rest of the body. Malcolm's heart had an ejection fraction of 10 percent. His heart had become big and dangerously weak, slowly, steadily stretching until it was a flimsy bag instead of a forceful pump.

I couldn't help but wonder why this had happened, especially since this kind of damage doesn't develop overnight. Most med students, residents, and Fellows feel the same way, naïvely asking the "Why?" questions over and over. We want to believe there are concrete answers to everything. But the attendings and the patients themselves remind us that, often, concrete answers don't exist. Heart failure can be the result of years of alcohol or drug abuse, but it can also come after a random encounter with a virus despite years of clean living. Sometimes there is another, benign cause that is normally treatable but once in a while becomes brutally destructive. Sometimes it's just unlucky genetics. There's a word for the cases with no apparent causes—*idiopathic*—but it is a fancy-sounding term for "nobody knows why." When these situations arise, all we doctors can do is clear our throats professionally and tell the patient and the family, "Mr. Jones, it seems you have idiopathic cardiomyopathy," and everyone nods as if that explains it.

In Malcolm's idiopathic case, the remaining 90 percent of unejected blood had pooled in his big, dilated ventricle, likely forming the blood clot that, through random bad luck, the weak, damaged ventricle had ejected into one of his coronary arteries. When the cath lab team had inserted the stent, they removed the immediate problem by opening the clogged artery and restoring blood flow. The coronary thrombus was gone, but Malcolm's heart remained weak, and with the left ventricle still pumping with pathetic inefficiency, the potential for another such clot was still there.

We've kept him alive so far. But just because Malcolm is in the cardiac intensive care unit doesn't automatically grant him a spot on the list for a new heart. He's here because the medications he's on and the type of IV hookup in his neck that measures pressures in and around the heart can only be done in the CICU. Our goal now is to stabilize him so that we can size him up: Is there a chance that he will recover? And if he doesn't, should we make the recommendation that he become a candidate for a new heart? Dr. James and I visit Malcolm every day and look for the signs, little and big, positive and negative, that might help us make this call. In particular, we watch for things that could keep him off the list, such as cancer, infection, kidney disease, or a serious pre-existing condition.

Although these decisions ultimately fall on the attendings, other key players get a chance to weigh in at the transplant meetings. Every Thursday at 3:00 p.m., a multidisciplinary team comprised of heart failure attendings, cardiac surgeons, nurses, nurse-practitioners, social workers, hospital insurance administrators, and Fellows gathers together to decide who makes the list—and who doesn't. These meetings are all about determining someone's fate, and they deal with every aspect of the transplant decision. (Even now, whenever I see that it's 3:00 on a Thursday, it still feels like "fate" time: Somebody is getting a spot on the heart list, or not.) They are candid, strictly off-the-record discussions of the patients, both those who have had the surgery and may be experiencing complications and those who are under consideration for a transplant. Altogether, only a handful of patients are considered per session. The conversations are not dramatic but businesslike and dry. If we do the operation, will the patient survive the surgery? And will he or she thrive afterward?

The focus of today's session is Malcolm. Should we list him? Should we delay? Before we get to the medical issues, there's another matter, a crass but real one.

Money. Heart transplants cost a fortune. Over an average of 30 days pretransplant through 180 days of procurement, hospital admission, physician treatment, and medications, a heart-only procedure costs $997,700, while a heart-lung combination costs $1,248,000. Harvesting the heart itself costs $80,000 (in case you've ever wondered what your heart is worth), and the immunosuppressant medications cost more than $30,000 per year. (Source: 2011 Milliman Research Report on organ and tissue transplants) Hardly any patient has that kind of money. Someone on the team has to make sure the patient has some form of adequate insurance, private or public, to cover it. Or the team member has to find a way to get the patient covered. This isn't a cold-blooded, protect-your-tail move on the hospital's part. It's a protect-the-patient's-tail move, so patients and their families don't spend the rest of their lives hounded by bill collectors and the law.

The hospital's insurance expert has already determined that Malcolm's insurance would not nearly cover the cost. But, as a veteran of this issue, she has a feel for whether she can get the coverage, and she is working with the state Medicaid office to see whether it could make up the shortfall. She gives Malcolm a tentative thumbs-up. If the patient qualifies, the team will do anything they can to make it happen. For now, Malcolm passes the money test.

Now to evaluate the hard factors (the medicine) and the soft factors (the patient's psyche, emotion, and acclimation). And in Malcolm's evaluation, something comes up: marijuana. The social worker reports that Malcolm had smoked marijuana about seven months prior. I'd been in the CICU when it was first noted. According to his recollection, Malcolm had taken a few tokes at a party over half a year ago. His cousin, who was visiting, corroborated the story, recalling that Malcolm had trouble inhaling without coughing.

The strict rule is, no drug use in the last six months, including cigarettes. Assessing the incident leads to a major discussion, and inadvertently becomes the social worker's moment in the spotlight. She launches into a sermon on the evils of drugs—all drugs, not just marijuana—and how his drug use should disqualify Malcolm. A doctor takes Malcolm's side. This was seven months ago, not six, so he's beyond the limit. The social worker says, "What if he's not telling the truth? What if he's taken drugs more recently?" The doctor counters that there is no indication of that. "He could have lied and said he's been a drug-free choirboy all his life, and we'd be listing him. Give him some credit for honesty. And the drugs have long been out of his system." She suggests he may have other undisclosed behaviors. A nurse comes to Malcolm's defense. Statistics are cited on both sides. Despite the clinical nature of the meetings, the human element always creeps in. We're making decisions that cross the line between medicine and morality, and people find Malcolm likable. We want him to have his chance.

Just when it seems the debate is going to go on indefinitely, the usually calm, unflappable Dr. James says, "For
God's sake, I smoked marijuana eight months ago and
haven't had a puff since." Several people snicker, since it's
doubtful he smokes marijuana at all, but it does bring the
discussion to an end.

But Malcolm still isn't on the list. There is another issue:
the abnormal CT scan of his chest, which could be the result
of fluid from heart failure or could indicate an inflammatory
condition. Either way, it raises the question of whether Malcolm's lungs are strong enough to survive surgery and support the transplant.

The pulmonologists' best guess is that Malcolm has inflammation in his lungs, perhaps due to pulmonary fibrosis,
a pre-existing condition of lung scarring thought to be potentially due to inflammation. So, we treat Malcolm pre-
sumptively: We decide to put him on steroids for pulmonary
fibrosis for two weeks and then get another CT scan.

The conclusion of the 3:00 p.m. Thursday meeting: Malcolm will not be on the heart transplant list. For now, he'll be
on the heart and lungs transplant list, because his own lungs
probably won't hold up under a heart-only transplant. The
heart and lungs list is like the Mega Millions lottery: Malcolm could win big but statistically he's on a worse list. Not
only does Malcolm have to survive this bout of heart failure,
possibly coupled with pulmonary fibrosis, but he also has to
get stronger. At the same time, we have to find a matching
heart and lungs, with the right blood type, and of the right
size. It's not every day that an Igloo cooler with a heart and
lungs shows up. And when and if it does appear, all of the
doctors—the cardiologist and the surgeon—have to agree, at

that point, that it's worth doing. Lungs are tough to transplant because they invariably get exposed to outside air and air is essentially poison when it comes to potential toxins and infections. Even clean mountain air carries potential microbiologic/toxin enemies that can wreak havoc on an immunosuppressed system—and Malcolm's lungs would be exposed to Baltimore's city air. Mega Millions odds.

As the weeks go by, I see Malcolm every day in the CICU, sometimes with Dr. James, sometimes on my own. He seems to be getting marginally better. Dr. James regards this small progress as significant. Now Malcolm can walk to the bathroom without stopping to rest, can say a few sentences without gasping. But is this improvement enough for an operation that would put him on the table for hours, detach his own cardiopulmonary system, and install someone else's?

Fortunately, Malcolm's next CT scan shows that his lungs look better after the steroids and heart medicine. This also means he might not need a heart-lung transplant, which makes a big difference when it comes to longer-term survival. Dr. James and I confer and decide. Ultimately, he goes on the heart transplant list—not the heart-lung list.

Although I see lots of patients, Malcolm is the one I keep thinking about. To remain stable, he needs to be on IV heart meds that can't be administered at home, so he's a prisoner of the ICU. At the next transplant meeting, the decision is made to put in an LVAD, a left ventricular assist device, which creates a pumping circuit that mimics and supplements what the left ventricle should be doing. Unlike a pacemaker, it doesn't jolt the heart; instead, it provides a continuous pumping action, like a rotor, enabling the left ventricle to work at an acceptable level. For Malcolm, this is good news and bad news. The good news is, with the device, he will be able to eventually go home. The bad news is that getting one reflects our concern that he might not get a heart transplant in time. An LVAD used to function exclusively as a bridge to a heart transplant, to get patients through what could be a two-year wait. But today, it's often put in instead of a transplant, as a destination therapy. No one knows which it will be for Malcolm, but it's apparent that his wait for a heart is going to be a long one.

Implanting the LVAD is a major operation that requires open-heart surgery: It splits the chest open, separates the rib cage, and is not unlike the physical trauma of a transplant. Recovery is tough. As patients often say, they feel as if they're going to "come apart." You have to relearn to sit up, and to hold a pillow to your chest when you cough. Malcolm is strong and has a good attitude, and he comes through re-markably well. The LVAD appears to be doing its job. Two weeks after surgery, we send Malcolm home, tethered to his power source, able to go out, but certainly not back to work. Given the timing of my rotation and the scarcity of hearts, chances are I won't directly care for Malcolm again.

That's another aspect of the job that's not right—not right for teaching or for treating—but I don't have a solution. Unless you're an attending cardiologist, seeing patients reg-ularly, you don't have ongoing doctor-patient relationships. As Fellows, we often see patients under the direst of condi-tions, sometimes near death; we diagnose and hopefully stabilize them; we send them home. And then the rest of their life happens, good or bad, and we often never know the long-term outcome. Did she live to be eighty-five? Or a week? Did she have more heart problems? Did she survive? Who treated her and with what? Did she die from an unrelated cause? Was she hit by a car in the supermarket parking lot? We don't know. For doctors in training, it creates a distance between doctor and patient, leaving us removed and perhaps less invested. They really aren't my patients; they're just temporarily under my care.

In some ways, I don't want to like Malcolm as much as I do—because there's some chance of a bad outcome, that he won't survive the transplant, or that he'll die waiting for a heart. If he does survive, for how long? Making rounds with Dr. James, I begin to understand that what appeared to be his disinterest in the average cases might be professional distance. You have to move on. There are always more patients, always more bad hearts.

Two days before my rotation ends, one patient, Mr. Graham, actually receives a transplant. I didn't treat him as a patient. In fact, I barely knew who he was, because he was one of the patients who waits at home, a name on a list until a heart is found. After a year, Mr. Graham has received word that there may be a heart for him, reason for both excitement and extreme caution. Plenty of patients have been called only to be told later that there was an issue with the donor heart—anything from developing arrhythmias prior to retrieval, to not pumping as vigorously as needed, or simply not looking strong enough to the surgeons. Because time is critical, the patient can't live more than two hours from the hospital. Donor hearts can be outside of the body for no more than six hours, so they generally come from nearby— Pennsylvania, Ohio, Delaware, and Virginia—by helicopter, ambulance, or airplane. Theoretically, you could get a heart from as far away as Florida in six hours, but any travel delay can irreversibly damage a donor heart that could have saved a life.

But Mr. Graham arrives at the hospital, his heart arrives, it's a go, and he has a successful operation. I see him in the surgical ICU a day later, and he appears to be doing all right, although *all right* is a relative term. He's tubed into and out of every imaginable place, wires connected, monitors beeping, fluids flowing, IVs dripping, tethered like a NASA astronaut. But his vital signs are stable, and there are no indications of organ rejection. Access to his room is restricted, since almost anything can do him damage during the critical recovery period. His family paces in the hallway, smiling, whispering into cell phones, nervous but happy. Their dad or granddad or uncle or brother has gotten a second chance . . . if it works. With only twenty or so of these operations in a year at an institution like Hopkins, the event creates a stir even among the most jaded doctors and nurses. Everybody is on high alert. Everybody wants success. We don't want to just do transplants; we want to do transplants that work.

When I finish the rotation, Mr. Graham's transplant is working. After that, who knows? Some other doctors will be there when Mr. Graham returns for his checkups, or with a rejection issue, or to adjust his meds, but not me. That's what's good and bad about the Fellow's role on the heart failure/transplantation rotation. It's intensely interesting, challenging, a chance to make a profound difference in a person's health at an intersection in time . . . but it is just that, an intersection, brief, random, and then over, disconnected from the person's longitudinal, lifetime care. Later in the year, I'll have another rotation on heart failure/transplantation, another "intersection," and perhaps that will give me a better idea of whether I could do what Dr. James does as my career. For now, as with Mr. Graham's outcome, who knows? Unlike Mr. Graham, I can put my fate on hold.

8

ROTATION: CARDIAC INTENSIVE CARE UNIT, PART I

The Other Hopkins

It's the middle of October. On to Cardiac ICU at Johns Hopkins's Bayview Medical Center. I'd like to say today is a crisp fall day with the leaves changing color, but I have no idea. I go from one sealed enclosure to another—hospital to car to home to car to hospital. I'm tired. I am also a little edgy going into this particular rotation. While I'd done cardiac intensive care unit rotations as a second- and third-year resident, this is my first time there as a Fellow, which means carrying greater responsibility for decisions. This time, I'm more doctor than student.

A few words about Bayview. Among medical residents and Fellows, Bayview carries a certain stigma. Although it's actually a newer facility, in many ways with better technological equipment and good staff, these are details that traditionalists like to ignore because it feels like a community hospital—a satellite, and not a clone. If Hopkins is the head-quarters, this is the branch office. A friend from my residency says, once you choose to train at Hopkins, you can find something wrong with just about anywhere else. We're taught state-of-the-art medicine by great attending physicians. We see the hospital ratings every year, and Hopkins keeps coming out on top. We go home exhausted every night, or morning, and figure the exhaustion was worth it. Our tolerance for anything else becomes low. We develop an elitist pride—exactly the kind of attitude that I don't want to have.

A practical difference between Hopkins "downtown" and Bayview is that many of Bayview's medical residents are just doing one year of internal medicine before going on to a different field, such as psychiatry, neurology, or ophthalmology. All of these specialties require a year of general internal medicine so that a psychiatrist can tell the difference between an anxiety attack and epilepsy. That's the good part. The downside is that part of my role as a CICU Fellow will be to make sure that, for example, the first-year psychiatry resident who correctly diagnoses a patient with mild depression doesn't happen to miss the patient's decompensated heart failure that is also present.

There's a sharp difference too in the way the patients are treated. Downtown, we are more aggressive about treating sick patients on non-ICU wards. We will move patients to the cardiac ICU when and if there is an emergency. At Bayview, the drill is to send the patient to the ICU first and ask questions later. As a Fellow on ICU, this can be frustrating when an ER doctor calls and says, "We're sending the patient to the ICU just to be safe. . . ." If one always followed the just-to-be-safe rule, all patients could be sent to the ICU because, technically, it is never absolutely possible to predict everything that could go wrong. Instead, you have to apply your medical knowledge and make a reasoned judgment. The fact is, between "take everyone to the ICU" and "take only the sickest to the ICU," there's probably an appropriate, wise middle ground.

Then there's the difference in patient population. Downtown is split between two extremes: international VIPs (Hollywood celebs, Wall Street moguls, Washington power brokers, European gentry, Saudi oil barons, coming to Hopkins for the best medicine) and the hospital's next-door neighbors (struggling families, single mothers, fatherless kids, drug sellers and users, urban casualties).

Bayview's constituency is somewhere between those two. The hospital is located geographically within the city limits, at the edge of Dundalk. It's a blue-collar/no-collar neighborhood, with a lot of second-generation Eastern Europeans, Poles, Greeks, Estonians, Latvians, Slavic diners and bars, and a Baltimore accent that can be almost unintelligible to outsiders. And that's a good description of one of my first Bayview patients a couple of weeks ago.

I'd been covering for another cardiology Fellow when I was asked to make the call on a larger-than-life character named Ray Jay. Ray was a forty-six-year-old, pony-tailed, busted-toothed contractor from the Highlandtown neighborhood. A heavy drinker and a red voter in a blue state, Ray cheered for the football team that he called the "Bawlamer Ravins." After a typical Friday night of gambling, cigarettes, and a few lines of cocaine, Ray had decided to check in to Bayview because of "weird" chest pains—caution that was completely out of character for Ray, who later revealed that when he broke his arm, he didn't go to the hospital until the next day, when his arm was bright blue and wouldn't move.

But by the time he got to Bayview on Saturday morning, Ray could barely walk without leaning on the wall. His EKG was abnormal, and his cardiac enzymes were slightly elevated and still rising. Ray had been taken to the cath lab, where we had found a tight blockage in his right coronary artery. What now? A decision had to be made, and the cath attending and the cardiac ICU attending decided it was time for the Fellow—me—to step into the real world and make the call.

Given Ray Jay's personal habits—cigarettes, cocaine, and general machismo—monitors, medicines, and watchful waiting is the cautious option. A stent might save Ray from a bigger heart attack, but the patient must take medications every day to keep it open. And Ray didn't seem to be someone who always acted in his own best interests. But after a short conversation in my head, I decide to take a chance on Ray. I explained to him that a stent could fix the blockage, but if he doesn't take his aspirin and clopidogrel—platelet-suppressing medications—he could clot off the stent and the whole artery could shut down, potentially bringing on a massive heart attack. "If we stent you and you snort coke, you're going to die. I promise you. Your call, Ray." He swears he'll be good. Of course, I wasn't sure whether to believe him. The cath team then stented him successfully. But for me, making the call myself was very different from observing and second-guessing someone else's decision.

Having met and treated Ray means that I feel as if I have a slightly better grip on this patient population. From the sixty-year-old former steelworker who has smoked two packs of Camels since the seventh grade to his reasonably healthy younger sister who eats a bag of Doritos every afternoon while watching her soaps, Bayview patients tend to be more of an American cliché. These patients come in with shortness of breath, or fluid in the lungs, or pain radiating down an arm, not because it's a world-famous hospital but because they're sick and Bayview is in their neighborhood.

The first week of cardiac ICU is stressful. After the initial day one, week one introductions to the nurses, techs, and attendings, the focus is on making rounds with the team, seeing patients, and getting used to the cardiac ICU routine. The nature of CICU is stress. Nothing unexpected may occur ... but it could at any time—the stress of potential stress.

I spend most of my time working with the residents, figuring out their quirks and foibles, who's good, who might panic, and who won't. Every night a resident is on call. If it's one you trust, you sleep. If it's one you don't, you're up all night with the pager dilemma. As the CICU Fellow, a quiet pager can worry me as much as a loud one. "What if they don't know when to call me? What if they don't recognize they need help? What if they're not relaying critical information?" My job is to prep the residents so they don't panic, so they do page me when they should and (preferably) not when they shouldn't.

I want to be a good teacher, and I know that the best learning takes place in the urgency of the moment, not just by watching but by doing. And that is one of the stresses I'm managing—that intersection of teaching and urgency, or clinical treatment. This first week, that's the toughest challenge for me—seeing things that need to be done now, knowing I could do them fast and right, whether it's a femoral central line or a central line into the chest or neck, yet knowing I have a responsibility to try to pass the knowledge on to someone else, but without heightened risk to the patient. So, I teach. It's stressful.

The stress is compounded by the fact that I am trying to be the teacher I would like to have as well. My attending for the first week is an excellent practitioner, but not an excellent teacher. And attendings need to be both. They need to know how to talk without being pedantic; to keep us interested; to question; to tease out our curiosity; to encourage but not allow a wrong conclusion; to make the case intellectually challenging, a Rubik's Cube we can solve; and to create a tutorial learning atmosphere. This particular attending is all about detail—sometimes germane, sometimes not—and not a natural teacher. At the first case presentations, he almost immediately interrupts the resident during her or his presentation. Rather than cutting in to point out where the resident's assessment is off or to contribute a relevant fact, he delivers an expansive footnote on exactly what the resident was saying, a minilecture on a point already made. Interrupting at the right time can be a great teaching technique. At the wrong time, it stops the momentum and undermines trust. Ideally, the residents should work their way through the potential scenarios, and find the answers on their own if possible—with the Fellow guiding and the attending providing an invisible safety net.

Still, letting the residents find their own way doesn't always pan out, as I learn after working with Pat. She's going to be a psychiatrist—and probably a good one, because she displays empathy, is smart, and can deal with me at my most impatient. One day, Pat tells me that she wants to learn to put in a central line. A central line (that is, a central venous line, also known as a central venous catheter, or CVC) is a catheter put into a large vein in the neck, chest, or groin, used to administer medication (such as vasopressors to treat critical hypotension), to get blood for tests, or to determine central venous pressure. Even with a topical anesthetic, the insertion can be painful. Wanting to learn such a delicate procedure is good, but on the other hand, it's unlikely that Pat will ever have to do it again in her career. There is a real, live patient who needs one. I've put in many CVCs, and in most situations, I can insert one in minutes. Pat is going to have to know all about compulsive behavior, Oedipal complexes, anxiety, schizophrenia, and bipolar disorder. But after this year, she'll never have to put a venous catheter into someone's neck. Am I doing the patient a disservice if I allow her to do this one? Would I want my mother to have a central line put in by a psychiatrist in training?

Still, I want to be a good teacher. Pat and I spend forty-five minutes setting everything up, prepping the patient, me prepping Pat. We even step outside the room for a rehearsal because I don't want the patient to hear me whispering instructions—"Okay, the next step is . . ."—and wonder, "Am I a lab rat?" I can't let Pat flail around, just bruising the patient's neck, and I need to give her a reasonable amount of time in which to try, whatever that means. How far should I let her go before stepping in? I wonder, why couldn't she say, "Hey, I'm going to be a shrink. You do it and I'll watch"? But she didn't. She asked to do it. And I don't want the lesson to be, "Don't bother to learn outside of your field." Instead, I find myself just wishing she weren't so earnestly interested.

We're gowned, in the room; the patient is comfortable that two good doctors are at his bedside, and I'm guiding Pat through it. To her credit, she's not too aggressive, the unintended by-product of overenthusiasm, and she's not too tentative, the result of first-time trepidation. So far, so good. But despite following the ultrasound pictures, she can't seem to get the needle into the blood vessel. I flex my fingers as if I had the line in them. I lean in, clench my teeth, and mimic the gesture of putting the line in. After her second and third attempts, I try hard not to say "No, let me." I have to loosen my grip on the reins. It isn't easy. But I know that others did so for me, and stay quiet.

The patient doesn't know there's a problem, but Pat does. After about twenty minutes, my mental time clock runs out. Calmly, professionally, so that the patient remains un- alarmed, I say, "I'll take it from here," which is academic code for "You're done. Give me the f—ing needle."

Within forty-five seconds, I have the needle in the vessel, the wire threaded, the catheter inserted along the guide wire, and the central line in—a relief. You don't want to take over and then struggle while the resident watches, nor do you want the patient to be the victim of two fumbled tries. (But you do mentally rehearse the failure speech to the resident, just in case. "This one was tougher than it looked. . . ." And you hope the resident doesn't think you're a pompous jerk. There are already enough of them in medicine.)

I can tell that Pat feels lousy. On the way out, I pull her aside and reassure her: "You did everything right. Your technique was good. Your pace was good. It was bad luck more than anything. It gets easier with time." I want her to feel better, but at best, she's going to feel less lousy. And she's probably not going to get better at it with time; she won't get enough practice. Having a basic understanding helps her as a doctor, no matter her specialty, to see the procedure in action, to know what it is, how it works, and when it's called for . . . just in case. But the reality is that she doesn't have to be good at doing it.

The next day, it's the end of week one. We do case presentations again, and again, the attending interrupts with minutiae. I think about how I've been teaching, how I've tried to be tolerant and gentle. I tried not to overlecture. But when I have to decide between letting the student fly the plane and taking the controls, I hear myself saying to Pat what I never wanted to hear as a student: "I'll take it from here." Is my approach better than the attending's or just different?

Fortunately, I am working with a different attending during the second week, Dr. Martin. I had worked with him for a few days back when I was a resident, so I know that he is a good diagnostician and clinician. Unusually, he also has a PhD in economics: While practicing cardiology full-time, he went to grad school at night because of his interest in health policy and the healthcare system as it relates to socioeconomic issues. And Dr. Martin has another intangible going for him: He's effortlessly cool. He doesn't try to seem young or hip; he's just a naturally appealing guy who is happy with himself and what he does every day—practice cardiology exceptionally well.

Rounding with him is like watching a virtuoso. Dr. Martin instructs more by example than by lessons, and his method is so low-key that it takes a while to realize that he is pulling the invisible puppet strings, gently guiding residents or Fellows to the right assumptions and decisions. But his strongest suit is his bedside manner. Communicating with patients and families is sometimes taken for granted in the high-tech world of today's medicine, but it's even more critical when the science involved can be so intimidating. Every doctor has to talk to families in sensitive situations. Most do it passably. Some overdo it and come across as too sensitive, over the top, like a bad movie actor. Some flip a switch— time to be sincere—and recite the script. But patients and families usually can tell the difference. Dr. Martin simply knows how to talk to people. He relates to the patients and their families, connecting with each one in a way that makes them all feel comfortable, no matter how dire the situation.

Case in point: I am at home late on Tuesday night when I get a call from the on-call resident about a patient coming into the CICU from the emergency room. Mr. Werdna, a retired plumber in his midsixties, was discovered by his wife, unresponsive, on the kitchen floor. When the ambulance arrived, the EMTs found the patient with no pulse, no gauge of how long he'd been down, without critical life signs, and with no apparent cause for the problem. The team intubated him "in the field"—that is, at home—and brought him to the nearest hospital: Bayview.

On the drive back to the hospital, I piece together what might have happened in order to get a sense of our options. Mr. Werdna may have had a primary cardiac arrest, which could have caused the loss of heart rate and drop in blood pressure. Or he might have had secondary arrest, due to a noncardiac event such as a seizure or stroke. In either case, during a critical time period, his heart was not delivering blood to vital organs, including his brain, and that may have done irreversible damage to one or more of those organs.

By the time I get to the hospital, his blood pressure and heart rate are improving. The twin goals are to keep him stable, with his systems running, and to put together a plan for his potential recovery. To try to fill in the blanks, I speak to his wife by phone. Mrs. Werdna is older than her husband by a good ten years, in her midseventies, evidently with poor vision and health issues of her own. In a shaky voice, she re-creates finding him, trying to rouse him, calling 911, the EMTs putting the tube in, and taking him away. She tells me he'd had a previous heart attack, and had been complaining of being tired the last few days but otherwise seemed all right. I try to convey the gravity of the situation to her, but over the phone there are no physical cues, so I can't tell if she understood or if she was still in denial or shock. I ask her to come in for a meeting, to prepare for what may be a negative outcome. Vulnerable families can't be expected to absorb an inundation of medicalspeak, so I put it in the plainest language I could: "He's our sickest patient in the cardiac intensive care unit." She says she will come in the next morning.

I stay overnight, help put in the central line and the arterial line, and get two hours of sleep in the on-call room. By morning I'm not looking or feeling too fresh, and I am in need of a shower and clean clothes. But I'm in no position to complain; the important thing is that we have managed to stabilize Mr. Werdna and that he is showing small signs of improvement. His blood work is improving, his kidney function gets better, and his elevated liver enzymes start to drop. His heart does not seem to have sustained catastrophic damage, which suggests that perhaps it wasn't his heart but possibly a seizure, some kind of aspiration, or a major neurologic event such as a stroke that caused his collapse.

There are less promising signs, though. Mr. Werdna is on a breathing machine without sedation. Normally, being on a breathing machine is both unnatural and uncomfortable. Having a tube in your throat is a decidedly unpleasant sensation; many patients thrash or open their eyes when they are intubated, necessitating the administration of sedatives for safety and comfort. But Mr. Werdna is showing no such physical responses—no jerking motions, nothing. And he has a continually low heart rate. This suggests that he might have an anoxic brain injury, which occurs when oxygen flow stops, starving the brain so it fails to perform. Hypoxic is partial oxygen deprivation; anoxic is total deprivation. The greater the deprivation, the worse the damage is to the brain, including potentially permanent loss of cognitive and physical skills. Recovery is possible but is determined by the brain parts affected, unpredictable at best, particularly at these early stages.

Dr. Martin comes in, and as the resident presents the case, I scrawl a little drawing on a scrap of paper. At the end, Dr. Martin asks what I think we should do. I hold up my rudimentary sketch of the brain. He nods. We aren't being irreverent. It's a picture of the situation; nothing else takes priority over the brain. And all of Mr. Werdna's organs seem to be recovering except his brain. I walk the team through a plan for the next twenty-four to forty-eight hours, explaining to the resident and the nurses that we have what appears to be perhaps an irreversible brain injury. Our job is to keep the brain alive and to give it its best chance at recovery under admittedly challenging medical circumstances. The other organs are secondary concerns at this point.

Afterward, I explain to Dr. Martin that I'd called the patient's wife the night before to set up a meeting for today; he agrees to join us. I meet Mrs. Werdna by the unit desk when she and her neighbors, who drove her, come in. I recognize her immediately—something about the catch in her gait, an older demeanor, and a frail voice. I go up to her, and her first question—"Is he getting better yet?"—makes it plain that she didn't fully comprehend our phone conversation. This makes a sit-down meeting—before she sees him with a tube in his lungs, IVs, a central line in his neck, electrodes on his scalp to monitor seizures—even more crucial. As I walk her down the hall, I make a combined medical and "neighborhood" diagnosis of how to deal with the situation. It isn't prejudice or gut; it's science. We turn into a small conference room and sit.

In the room are Dr. Martin and the CICU nurse, along with Mrs. Werdna, her neighbors, and me. I begin, "Mrs. Werdna, when we talked last night, I threw a lot of information at you, so I think we should go over it." I can tell she doesn't want to hear it; she knows it's bad. Meanwhile, Dr. Martin is watching me to see how I handle it. He mentioned before the meeting that he wanted me to start by setting the stage very realistically. Mrs. Werdna's husband is not likely to recover. With severe neurologic injury, the best he can hope for is to remain on life support for a few days. She's trembling, and I start to worry that she may fall apart. I go slowly, but not too slowly, because I don't want to drag it out. "Your husband is very sick, critically ill." I let my words sink in and then say, "We're providing him with life support right now. When you see him, he's going to be hooked up to a lot of equipment." I purposely use terms such as *critically ill* and *life support,* and I look for comprehension in her face.

In fact, Mr. Werdna had not suffered a massive heart attack (as his cardiac enzymes have returned to normal levels). The unhappy truth is that Mr. Werdna's body and brain had already begun to die on the kitchen floor, a process that was interrupted only temporarily by the paramedics. The body has remarkable resilience, an ability to recover in almost every organ system—lungs, kidneys, liver, even the heart. The one organ that begins to die quickly, with little chance of bouncing back, is the brain. And blood flow to Mr. Werdna's brain had been cut off for five or more minutes—the danger zone.

When his wife asks, "Is he awake at all?" I know she's beginning to understand. I tell her, no, he probably won't know that she's in the room. Then she asks the inevitable—what happened and why. What did I do? He was fine two days ago. What should I have done? The bottom line is, we don't really know. I tell her, "What we know, based on the testing in the last eighteen hours, is that he's a man with serious medical problems, and people like that can get very sick, very quickly." More important, I add, "Sometimes there aren't clear warning signs. You didn't miss something. It isn't your fault." Dealing with the likelihood of his death is enough; there's no reason she should be blaming herself. Her friends listen and hold her hands. Though only in their fifties, they aren't pictures of health themselves. Mrs. Werdna's support team seems as weak as she is, gathered for a vigil over the one who'd, at least to them, seemed the strongest.

Dr. Martin, who has been quietly monitoring the scene, leans forward now and looks at Mrs. Werdna. "Sweetheart, how are you holding up?" Her face says, "As well as I can." He goes on: "I have to tell you, we doctors are not miracle workers. There are some questions we don't know the answers to." With these plain phrases, he resets her expectation levels to reality. We don't have all the answers. Sometimes there are no answers. He then reiterates the medical plan. "As Dr. Muñoz said, at this point we're most concerned with his brain because he went too long a time without oxygen to the brain." The choice of words, "too long," was again simple but strong, perfect communication, so subtle an outsider might miss it. The last thing we want to do is provide false hope, nor should we label a tragedy prematurely.

I'm taking mental notes on every nuance. This is not something med school, residencies, or fellowships necessarily teach. Our time is filled cramming knowledge and experience into us, and little is left for human subtleties. We're supposed to pick them up on our own, which means that some people never do. I've seen academically brilliant colleagues who talk to patients and families as if they were spouting data into a digital recorder. "This is stage IV melanoma. There are treatments but no cure. Expected survival is from four to thirteen months. . . ." Arguably, it cannot be taught. Either you're someone who is sensitive to people or you aren't. That's why when you come across a Dr. Martin, you know you should pay attention. We're here to treat people, not charts.

Mrs. Werdna asks Dr. Martin if her husband is in pain. He leans in, speaks softly, slowly, and compassionately, and puts his hand on hers. "I can tell you, he is not. Your pain is far greater than the pain he feels. I know you hurt right now." Her husband is not suffering. Because his brain is not working properly, it will not allow him to sense pain. Dr. Martin conveyed all that without relying on cold medical words. I am blown away. I've never heard another doctor communicate this way.

Mrs. Werdna looks at Dr. Martin and gets teary but doesn't break down: She is physically frail, but rock solid in character. Then she says something that I've heard before, but that always amazes me. She thanks us. We've just told her that her husband is hanging on to life by a kite string, and that his brain has likely already let go. But she says, "Thank you all for everything you're doing for him. He couldn't be in better hands." Families invest their confidence in our medical knowledge, but evaluate us on our ability to connect. If you can connect, you're a good doctor. If you can't, you aren't. It isn't rational, but it's not crazy either. Oftentimes, patients and family members can gauge only the human elements. Do you hear me? Can you feel my distress? Do you care? Mrs. Werdna says she and her husband couldn't be in better hands, an opinion that is largely based on Dr. Martin's communication skills, not actual proof of his clinical ability. In theory, we could all be mediocre. But that's what a lot of good medicine is about—reaching the patient or family so you can practice good medicine. If the adage "Ninety-five percent of success is showing up" is true, the medical corollary is, "Ninety-five percent of being a good doctor is the ability to look the patient in the eye." I am not ashamed to say I will try to memorize what Dr. Martin said, how he said it, his pauses, even his facial expressions. He is a master at this, and this is one of the most indelible lessons of my career.

After the meeting, we guide Mrs. Werdna and her friends to her husband's room. Dr. Martin backs out: "I want to give you time to yourselves. We're just down the hall outside if you need anything." She sits by her husband, but in reality, she's alone. He's not there anymore. I stay a few more minutes, then leave. An hour later, I see the neighbors escort her out.

At the next meeting about Mr. Werdna, I set the plan. We'll wait a day on the remote chance things might improve, but our next meeting with Mrs. Werdna will almost inevitably involve telling her that her husband isn't going to make it. Dr. Martin says only, "Sadly, I agree," which surprises me a bit. From someone as understated as he is, that brief comment is a vote of confidence.

In the ensuing hours, Mr. Werdna's organ systems improve but his brain does not. He's just not waking up, although he occasionally exhibits jerking, seizure-like movements, episodes that are understandably troubling and confusing to his family. We speak to the neurologists involved to help manage these sporadic movements, but they are most likely the result of faulty electrical firings in his injured brain. It's now Thursday, two and a half days after Mr. Werdna was admitted. He displays no primitive reflexes, but he is not technically "brain-dead." His brain waves have not flatlined. His jerking motions show up as little blips on his EEG (electroencephalogram). But his chances for recovery are as close to zero as you can get. All of this brings up another major medical dilemma: At what point does keeping a patient alive because there is a very small chance then cross over into keeping the patient alive when there is no hope? There isn't a specific moment in time—say, day two at 11:15 in the morning—when a patient's fate is sealed. There's no test that says, as of right now the brain will never recover. The judgment isn't black-and-white; it evolves from gray.

I call Mrs. Werdna and tell her that it would be good for us to meet tomorrow: It is time for us to deliver our verdict. We could keep her husband alive attached to life support, but there is virtually nothing we can do to change his neurologic fate or make him better. Some families ask, "Does this mean he'd be hooked up forever?" We say, "Yes." And they often say, "He wouldn't want that." This leads to a discussion of withdrawal of care (i.e., ventilator). And because some people die not in seconds or minutes, but in hours or days following that step, I want the family to fully understand the situation. I also ask Dr. Young, a second-year resident from Hopkins who is on-call that night, to attend the meetings as well. I want the family and friends to recognize her as a familiar face. If Mr. Werdna should die on her watch, in the middle of the night, that 1:00 a.m. phone call shouldn't come from a total stranger.

Unlike our last meeting, this one has no rehearsal. We arrange ourselves around Mrs. Werdna, with Dr. Martin and the nurse sitting opposite her and her neighbors. Dr. Young sits at one end of the table, and I sit at the other. I summarize our earlier talk and then say, "Now, I've got to tell you that we don't have good news." I pause, just as Dr. Martin did, to let this sink in. Whenever he says something highly consequential, he stops to allow people to digest and process it. He knows that nothing we say in the next ten seconds will be heard, not after that. I wait, then go on. "Despite everything we have done to support and comfort your husband, to take the best care of him we know how, whatever brought this on has caused a severe injury to his brain." That's a lot to absorb—despite support, comfort, care, injury to his brain. Again, I wait for Mrs. Werdna's recognition and continue. "With the help of our neurology doctors—the brain specialists—and with our own experience, we can tell you that his brain is not going to get better . . . ever." Mrs. Werdna is teary but does not break down. I try to channel Dr. Martin by holding Mrs. Werdna's hand as I go on. "One thing I can assure you is you are all in far greater pain than anything Mr. Werdna is experiencing right now. He is not in pain. He's not suffering." Dr. Martin is there, and although I have appropriated his speech almost verbatim, he is fine with it. The unspoken message is: This is what I teach. It works. Take it; use it.

Through her tears, Mrs. Werdna says, "I want you all to know how much I appreciate everything you've done." She pauses, then says, "I understand he's not going to get better." Her neighbors nod. She asks, "What am I supposed to do?" She literally does not know what to do. Who does? Who has had experience with such things? Neither she nor I have ever been in this circumstance before. Despite my calm demeanor, I'm still struggling to respond when Dr. Martin says, "I agree with everything Dr. Muñoz has said. We are heartbroken and terribly sorry that you are dealing with this, that your husband has gotten sick in a way that he's not going to get better . . . that he's never going to wake up." That last phrase, "never going to wake up," gives finality to the scene. It's no longer when or maybe or probably; it's "never."

And "wake up" is the perfect, most empathic way to express this because it evokes sleeping rather than death. It is an easier image to deal with. "As Dr. Muñoz said, he isn't suffering, doesn't feel pain. The part of him that made him who he was, that was your husband for all those years, that man is gone. That part of him is in a better place now." I know that I don't have enough lines in my face to pull off the phrase "in a better place now." But Dr. Martin has invoked it to imply that Mrs. Werdna's husband has moved on, and now she can too. His words also free her from guilt, in case she's not in the room at the moment he dies. Even though his heart is beating, he's already gone. Dr. Martin has broken terrible news to Mrs. Werdna, given her permission to let go of her husband, and to do so without guilt, with simple and heartfelt phrases.

Where is the line between hope and hopeless? It's blurred. The moment of profound change is clear only in retrospect, if then. After twenty-four hours? Forty-eight? Three months? Our job is not just about administering medicine; it's also about managing expectations and treating the patient and the family, enabling them to accept the end. Some parts of the world make it simpler, empowering someone at a hospital to say, "It's over." But that's not the way we do it here, at least right now. We do it case by case, doctor by doctor. And not all doctors are Dr. Martin.

When families can't let go, technology can prolong the demise of a loved one at staggering emotional and financial costs. We possess the scientific ability to keep someone alive. But the cost of maintaining a person in that state indefinitely is in the millions, to say nothing of the emotional costs. Sometimes families choose to do so for reasons of denial, or religious beliefs, or misunderstanding, or simply because they feel they have no right to "kill" someone who is alive, even if only artificially. And there isn't a lot we can do to stop it. That's why Dr. Martin is so impressive. He doesn't take away the family's prerogatives, nor does he fuel false hopes. He presents reality in a way that enables them to let go.

Dr. Martin then lays out the process for Mrs. Werdna. "Everything will happen at your pace and timing. Now that we know he's not going to wake up, we can disconnect some of the machines to create a more peaceful place, a little less beeping and buzzing. We can leave the room and you can visit with him by yourself, at peace. Some families prefer a day or two. . . ." It's clear that Mrs. Werdna is beginning to grasp the reality of her situation and accept the outcome. Nodding slowly, she says, "Doctor, you said he's not going to wake up. I trust you. We don't need any more time. I don't want to drag it out. I just want him to be comfortable." She turns to the neighbors. They all nod in agreement. She asks for a few moments alone with her husband, then says she'd like a chaplain to come in for a prayer. Then she thanks us again. We step into the hall. I notice that the resident, Dr. Young, is teary. She turns to me. "That was the most incredible family meeting I've ever seen. How do you guys know how to do that?" I shake my head. The fact is, I learned most of what I know in the last three days from watching Dr. Martin.

Our next step is to remove the life-support machinery. We have the staff shut down most of the scientific "noise"— the alarms and monitors—around Mr. Werdna and take the breathing tube out so he'll look more familiar to his wife.

The only equipment we leave is an EKG, because it will tell us when his heart stops beating. The staff also remakes the bed with a fresh blanket and pillows. The formality and the lack of medical clutter often help families say goodbye with dignity.

Mr. Werdna's heart stops beating about fifteen minutes after care is formally withdrawn. The ICU nurse is the first to know it via the monitor at her station. She alerts me and the resident and asks me to pronounce him. Technically, Mr. Werdna isn't dead until I have listened to his heart for a minute to ensure that there are no extra beats, watched him not breathe, and then written a confirming note in the chart. To me, these steps seem nonsensical, especially now, when the patient is unquestionably dead. I'm supposed to put a stethoscope on his chest as if I were listening for something that obviously isn't there, which is cruel, since the families will reflexively hope for the impossible. A family member might ask with a tone of confusion and irrational hope, "What do you hear? What are you listening for?" I see Mrs. Werdna sitting right there, next to the bed, and I decide to sidestep the macabre ritual. I don't touch the body or examine it. Instead, I look at the monitor at the station, see the flat line, then look at the EKG strip to confirm that it too is flat. The resident is watching when I pronounce Mr. Werdna officially dead: "He has passed. Time of death, 2:17 p.m." Sometimes, following a protocol is not the right thing to do. Dead is dead. Worry about the living, the family. To me, this was the better way to do it.

*   *   *

One case. One doctor. One career moment. But these moments are something you have to keep in perspective. They're rare. You can't let the big moments overshadow everyday doctor work, or you'll compromise your ability to deal with the average crisis. The CICU is full of serious cases, but we're supposed to treat them all with the same gravity. The reality is, you have only so much emotional capacity. If a daughter says, "My father is light-headed," you may think, "He'll be fine; it's probably nothing." But it's not fine or nothing to her or her father. You have to resist your own reflexes. It's our job to separate these special moments from the everyday, but it's counterintuitive.

You can't walk out of a powerful end-of-life encounter and into the CICU to a patient who is sick, but not at death's door, and treat her in an offhand or casual way: This is what I tell myself as I walk in to see a sixty-two-year-old woman with heart failure due to valvular disease. What she has is not immediately life-threatening, but she's scared. We can medicate her and she'll be okay. But she doesn't know that. She thinks she could die. I talk. I explain. I listen. I read her signals. Am I getting through the way Dr. Martin did or even the way I did with Mrs. Werdna?

Throughout the next two weeks, I consciously invoke my mantra "Move on to the next patient. Focus. Move on to the next. Focus. . . ." I want to treat all of these cases as important, not just the out-of-the-ordinary ones. But there's the community hospital challenge of case mix. Plenty of people in the Bayview CICU (despite its name—cardiac *intensive care* unit) just aren't that sick. You can move patients out of the unit once they're ready for a regular medical floor, but you can't control the inflow, the ones the ER doctors put there "just in case." Hence the occasional Fellow's crack, "Just saw a guy in the unit who's in better shape than I am." During the last week of the rotation, I see seven to ten patients a day, all told about forty-five patients. Two get stents. Two have open-heart procedures. Six are transferred to floors where they belong. Two die in the unit. Some are still there when I leave. I'm being a cardiologist—the day-to-day routine of practicing.

When I am away from the hospital, I try to put it in perspective, a hierarchy of what's most important, what's less so. I can never do it when I'm there. I run in the mornings and have conversations in my head. Did I handle that case right? Did the resident? What would I do differently next time?

On Friday, the final day of the rotation, Dr. Martin stops me in the hall for an end-of-rotation talk. He asks, "How do you think things have gone these last two weeks?" I don't answer quickly, remembering how he uses waiting to make sure to say the right thing. "Dr. Martin, I'm not a sunshine blower or a yes-man, but I want to tell you that I really appreciate your approach. . . ." I detail what I've learned, how his methods and style of communication made the rotation more significant, how it all made me a better Fellow, and how I want to challenge myself further as a result. When I finish, he's surprisingly effusive: "Dan, you get it. You understand the complexity. You're going to be very good with people. In fact, you already are." He goes on, "The house staff likes working with you, and you're well respected." Then he offers, "If there's anything I can do to help you in your career, I want to do it." Medical training doesn't have many moments such as this. Usually, it's all classrooms, labs, clinics, charts, patients, and treatments—and being congratulated by one of the greatest teachers I've met so far is a meaningful moment for me.

This rotation opened my mind about Bayview and about drawing conclusions in general—both thanks to Dr. Martin. Here's a physician who had world-class training and who then chose to practice at Bayview. And he practices very good medicine here. Just when I had all my prejudiced notions about how the branch office couldn't measure up to the "real Hopkins" neatly in place, I end up having probably my best rotation experience. Lesson: Don't make a diagnosis until you get all the information. I'll carry it with me.

Another lesson I will take with me is the experience of latitude Dr. Martin gave me in managing the team—teaching, directing residents and nurses, laying out patient assessments, treatment plans, family communication. On rounds, at the end of each resident presentation, he'd invite me to lead: "Dr. Muñoz, what would you like to do here?" He was always supportive. If he did add something substantive, he'd low-key it—"And you might consider this . . ."—never taking credit. It was as if I were the attending, except I had a great attending to back me up. To turn the cliché around, I was performing with a net, a very good net.

This is also the first rotation that has given me a hint of the kind of work concentration I might want long-term. I like CICU challenges, the pace, the range of cases, the doctor-patient interaction, not just scans and readouts but doctor to patient, plus the element of teaching. Is this a glimpse of my future? We'll see.

9

ROTATION: ELECTROPHYSIOLOGY

Circuit Board of the Heart

Another rotation finished, another one beginning. Last Friday, I was deep into the human side of cardiology—people with heart problems. Today, I'm back in the tech world, starting a rotation in EP—electrophysiology. It's one of the sharpest contrasts in the fellowship, exceeded only by following consults (all about patients) with nuclear (all about pictures).

EP is the electrical study of the heart—in the vernacular, doctor as electrician. Commonly, you see an electrophysiologist for a pacemaker or defibrillator, but there's considerably more to it. The heart is a muscle, but it's also a highly choreographed electrical symphony, sending out impulses, which, when unsteady, cause short circuits. If there's any heart rhythm disturbance—an irregular electrical signal that causes symptoms or potential danger—it often requires evaluation by an EP (electrophysiologist).

The parameters of an arrhythmia (abnormal rhythm) are expansive. There are two clinical subsets: "bradyarrhythmias" and "tachyarrhythmias." Bradyarrhythmia, or bradycardia, is a heartbeat that is slow, sixty beats per minute or less, usually because of blocking of electrical impulses in the heart's conduction system—simply put, wiring gone bad. There are trained Olympic athletes or some young, very fit people who have very slow resting heart rates. But in an ordinary person, if the rate falls below fifty beats per minute, symptoms such as fainting, shortness of breath, dizziness, light-headedness, chest discomfort, palpitations, and possibly death can occur.

Tachyarrhythmia, or tachycardia, is a heartbeat that is inappropriately fast, usually over one hundred beats per minute in an adult. If the heart rhythm is too rapid, it means the heart is in overdrive, working unsustainably hard. The heart may not have enough time to fill during ventricular relaxation (that is, the time span between contractions) and may pump an inadequate amount of blood to the brain or body. In certain vulnerable patients with little to no reserve, the immediate result can be serious: hypotension (low blood pressure) and a dangerous compromise in perfusion of vital organs (that is, delivery of sufficient flow to feed and support the organs, particularly the brain). The eventual result can be worse: organ failure or death. The job of the electrophysiologist is to identify and determine which of those heart rhythms is relevant and potentially dangerous, and what needs to be done.

Of all the rotations, this one feels the most foreign to me, the most daunting, because the people who typically do EP have intimidating intelligence. EP doctors tend to be electrical engineering majors, the type who never left their dorm rooms and whose senior theses had brilliant, incomprehensible titles. EPs have to be part physicist, part engineer, part biologist, part wizard, and able to integrate all of those roles. Plenty of cardiologists, if they're honest, would likely admit to not comprehending the pure science behind electrophysiology. And at this point in my training, my exposure to the management of funky heart rhythms has been modest—the term *funky* itself a dead giveaway.

Fortunately, in electrophysiology, you have a lot of bosses. Instead of one principal supervising attending for the entire rotation, you have one per week, over four weeks. Part of my job as a first-year Fellow is to carry the EP consult pager, which means that I will be acting as the first line of contact. A typical call on the EP-1 pager could be an issue with a patient on another service (hospital department) who has a pacemaker and the team wants to know if it's working properly. Simple, straightforward stuff. Except that I don't know what is or isn't working right, even though it is my job to try to decipher what the heart rhythm is, what I think needs to be done, and then hand the case off to a senior EP Fellow or the EP attending. It strikes me as perversely funny that when other doctors anywhere in the hospital have an EP-related question, they will call me—like giving a kid those plastic airplane captain's wings and saying, "Go fly the plane." I have nothing to qualify me except my official EP-1 pager.

My first EP consult call comes in at 10:00 a.m., when the resident on one of the medicine service teams leaves me a message: "We admitted this guy overnight with an abnormally slow heart rhythm. We've got to know, does he need a pacemaker?" This is exactly the kind of scenario I feared: A doctor is asking something I know precious little about, and it's important. So I do what any prudent person would. I call the resident and say, "I'm happy to see the patient. Thanks for the consult. Get back to you shortly," which is code for "I don't know yet, but I will." In other words, I stall.

I'm not worried about coming up with the right answer. There are places I can look: textbooks, journals, published guidelines. There are people I can ask: the EP experts. I'm concerned about sending a message of uncertainty to the doctors and perhaps to the patient or the patient's family. And the best remedy for temporary ignorance is immediate diligence, to overdo the digging and learning, and get smart. Fortunately, my approach is possible because the pace of EP is generally measured and sane. My pager is not beeping like a broken car alarm. There's plenty of time to ask questions, review the medical literature on the subject, and ultimately confer with the attending. Whereas general cardiac consults can be a much faster-paced rotation, with less time available to "look it up" when you don't know the answer, the EP consult caseload tends to be slow and painstaking, like untangling marionette strings.

According to the chart, the patient is a seventy-seven-year-old man. My initial impression from the door is that he looks uncannily like Blue, the elderly frat member from the movie *Old School*. Our Mr. Blue lives in a little apartment complex, with neighbors and friends who look after him, but he's fairly independent for his age. He was brought to the hospital by an EMS (emergency medical service) team after a neighbor found him dizzy and light-headed, unable to get out of bed or walk without almost falling over. The ER doctors immediately noted that his heart rate was thirty-five rather than in the normal sixty to eighty range—and Mr. Blue was no Olympic decathlete. At his age, a heart rate of thirty-five could be a life-threatening emergency, but what matters most is whether his heart is generating enough perfusion. The way to find out is not that complicated: "Sir, how are you feeling?" If his only answer is a moan, it's a clear indication his brain is not being adequately perfused. If he can look you in the eye and says, "Doc, I'm fine. The ambulance brought me in because I haven't been feeling so hot," that's a temporary confirmation that, for the moment, his brain is getting adequate blood flow.

Fortunately, the resident reports that Mr. Blue is able to converse. His blood pressure is okay, about 120 over 70. More important, he's awake, alert, and seems oriented to the place, time, and situation. He's passed the superficial tests. Nonetheless, somebody who's seventy-seven with a heart rate of thirty-five doesn't get sent home even if he is clinically perfusing. Instead, Mr. Blue is admitted to the cardiac step-down unit, which acts as an intermediary stage between a regular floor and the CICU. There, a first look at Mr. Blue's EKG reveals some amount of heart block, or in EP terms, a degree of "conduction abnormality between the top chambers and the bottom chambers."

There are three basic degrees of heart block. First-degree block is less serious, and it will appear on the EKG as a prolonged interval between the first and second wave of the cardiac cycle: a delay that shouldn't be there but may cause no immediate harm. A lot of people live asymptomatically with first-degree heart block. Second-degree heart block is the fuzzy area, a slightly more abnormal conduction pattern, between the relatively benign first and highly threatening third degrees. Third-degree, or complete, heart block, is when the top chambers and the bottom chambers aren't coordinating activity. A patient in complete heart block will usually end up in the CICU, a wire placed through a catheter in the neck, floated down into the heart, to send electrical impulses to control the heart rate until a permanent pacemaker can be safely implanted.

It appears that Mr. Blue belongs to one of the subsets of second-degree heart block. Since he had a normal EKG at Hopkins a year prior, this situation is new and not good. And this is why the internal medicine team has asked for a consult on whether Mr. Blue needs a pacemaker.

Before I see Mr. Blue, I do a "chart biopsy," which is an objective look inside the patient based on his or her total records—what's happened, what's been done, patient history, as well as the computer data on lab work and tests. I do it as a matter of practicality, a pattern I got into during cardiology consults. Walking in uninformed and asking the patient to tell me about himself would result in a conversation that could last for hours and never reveal what I need to know. The reality is that my task is not to hear a life journey, but instead to focus on developing an understanding of the patient's heart rhythm. Based on Mr. Blue's records, his bedside chart, and EKGs, I confirm that it looks to be a subset of second-degree heart block. At the nurses' station, I scan the monitors on all the patients, and see that, thanks mostly to the passage of time, Mr. Blue's heart rate is now forty, at least up from thirty-five.

When I walk in, Mr. Blue is lying in bed, a happy, smiling

guy who has no idea why so many doctors are interested in him. I start off by introducing myself and asking some basic questions. "What brought you to the hospital?" He says, "Well, I felt a little funny at home, but now I feel better, and to tell you the truth, I don't know why I'm here." I ask, "Is anything bothering you?" He answers almost before I finish. "Yup! I'm hungry." In the med school course informally titled Figuring Out Fast Whether the Patient Is Sick, if the chief complaint is hunger, it's usually a good sign.

Then I start to ask more focused questions. Instead of asking "How long have you had health issues?" or "Has a doctor ever told you before that you have second-degree heart block?" I ask whether Mr. Blue has ever passed out before, and whether he often feels dizzy or light-headed. I ask direct questions about chest pain, shortness of breath, as symptom-based as possible. His answers are generally in the negative. He's independent and functional, able to walk a few blocks every day without the assistance of a walker or a cane. He's a content retired guy. But he does acknowledge that in the last two weeks, he's had a couple of episodes where, during mild exertion, walking upstairs or getting out of bed, he felt light-headed. The most pronounced episode was yesterday, the day he came in.

Coupling this with his heart rhythm, I begin to wonder if Mr. Blue has deteriorated to second-degree heart block in just the last three weeks. If that were the case, he might need a pacemaker, which would assure his heart rate wouldn't fall below a critical threshold (fifty beats per minute, for example), and he wouldn't get symptomatic again. But it's my first EP consult, in my first week of EP rotation, so I'm wary.

To qualify for a pacemaker, a patient must be diagnosed

with a heart rhythm issue that is causing his or her symptoms and that has no underlying cause that we might be able to correct or reverse. In Mr. Blue's case, he has a heart rhythm issue, which is causing his symptoms and which doesn't seem to be something that we can quickly correct. I know that because I looked for other culprits—specifically, his medications. Mr. Blue is taking beta-blockers, which are prescribed to slow the heart rate and control the blood pressure. Too much beta-blocker and the heart can slow excessively. But this man has been on the same dosage of a beta-blocker for high blood pressure and coronary disease for years. The effects of a wrong dose would have declared themselves long ago. I check his liver and kidney function, because sometimes abnormal liver or kidney function can impact how the body metabolizes a beta-blocker, causing it to build up in the system and act like a higher dose than it is. But Mr. Blue's liver and kidney function are both fine.

Nonetheless, while he's in the hospital, we stop his beta-blocker in order to prevent his heart rate from slowing even further. I don't expect that decision will correct his heart rhythm and obviate the need for a pacemaker, but this is my first consult and I err on the side of exploring options before electing to implant the device.

That evening, I meet with the week's EP attending, Dr. Harry, and summarize the consult: "My sense is this is symptomatic bradycardia with second-degree heart block in the absence of a clearly reversible cause of that bradycardia. Because he is symptomatic, it's an indication for a pacemaker." He nods, so I go on: "In the interim, we've held back his beta-blocker because his heart rate's thirty-five to forty." Dr. Harry talks to the patient himself, then concludes, "I agree with your assessment, but let's give him a day or two more off his beta-blocker and see what happens."

The next day when I walk in, Mr. Blue's heart rate is up to fifty, which is still low but considerably better. He remains hungry but otherwise has no complaints. The nurse takes him for a walk around the unit with a monitor on—no panting or wheezing, no pain—and he gets his heart rate up to the low seventies, which is very close to normal. When he lies down and is at rest, it dips back to the high forties to fifty, but still trending in the right direction. This puzzles me: Our only intervention so far has been stopping Mr. Blue's beta-blocker. Why is he getting better when we withhold a medication he's been taking for years? And if he *is* getting better, is he no longer a candidate for a pacemaker? It's good news, but it doesn't make physiologic sense, at least not to me.

My instincts say, do some medical detective work. It turns out the patient's neighbor, a nursing student, helps with his medications. I get her on the phone and tell her that one of Mr. Blue's medications may have caused a problem but we can't figure out why. Before I can get another sentence out, she says, "I'm glad you called, because I've been concerned about his medicines for a long time. I try to lay them out, keep them in order, but now he's less able to distinguish between the pills. I worry he gets confused, taking not enough of one, too much of another." If her instincts are right, there's a real possibility that Mr. Blue's low heart rhythm was a response to accidentally taking too much of the beta-blocker.

The next day, after another twenty-four hours without the beta-blocker, Mr. Blue's heart rate is in the low sixties. By the third day, it's up to the midsixties, and he has a normal heart rhythm. The second-degree heart block is gone. Mr. Blue was discharged the next day, four days after being admitted—with a better pill-taking system in place, but without a pacemaker.

This is a humbling first consult because it makes me realize that my initial assessment was far too preliminary. The treatment plan quickly evolved from "Second-degree heart block, heart rate of thirty-five, serious symptoms, put in a pacemaker" to "No major problems, no light-headedness, no shortness of breath, just hungry, pretty soon we can send him home." The "intervention" ended up being a very different variety than what I, or even the EP attending, Dr. Harry, originally thought we would need to do. It didn't involve putting anything in; it involved finding out the patient was unintentionally taking too much beta-blocker. Sometimes waiting is good medicine, and Dr. Harry had the wisdom to weigh the possibilities before acting. And I'm glad that I followed my instincts, that I also trusted my doubts were trying to tell me something. Mr. Blue is a classic example that a lot of medical problems are due to a lack of information—information that may not be immediately available from the patient . . . but that doctors can obtain if they have the time, the resources, and the inclination to do a little digging.

The rest of the patients I see during the rotation are mostly the quick in and out, like patients with atrial fibrillation, who are in for electrical cardioversions. Atrial fibrillation, or atrial flutter, occurs when the top chambers of the heart are whipping away at too fast a rate. The bottom chambers that pump the blood try to ignore some of the noise from the top, but can't and end up with a random, overly noisy beating of the heart that can cause symptoms such as shortness of breath, palpitations, and angina. Almost any exertion results in exhaustion, or the classic patient description of "I feel crappy." Because the EP doctors specialize in mapping out the electrical network of the heart like a schematic diagram of house wiring, they can try to burn certain areas in an attempt to break the short circuits and get rid of the electrical impulse causing the abnormal rhythm. Cardioverting the patient, or directing an electrical current into the chest, can get the patient back into a normal or sinus rhythm, often improving or relieving symptoms and heart function.

My job is to meet the patients in a preprocedure room and talk to them, review their records, go through the consent procedure, where I describe what we're going to do, cover the risks and benefits, and get their permission to proceed. Then I page the attending to room 11, the procedure room, to obtain the official go-ahead. We sedate the patients so they're asleep but not "fully under," while having them hooked up to monitors to track their vital signs—blood pressure and oxygenation. Once the patients are sedated, we put pads on their chest and administer timed delivery of electric shock, to reset the cardiac cycle. Again, with the go-ahead from the attending, I press a button that unleashes a two hundred–joule shock to the patient's chest. For the next second, everyone holds their breath to see if it put the heart back in normal rhythm. Despite being sedated and asleep, patients will occasionally let out a bloodcurdling shriek or string of profanity after being whacked in the chest by all that electricity. Fortunately, the sedating medications ensure that patients do not remember this, and once the sedation wears off, most leave the same day.

But things can and do go wrong. In any delivery of electricity, there's a mathematical chance of inducing a faster or more unstable rhythm, and that can be life-threatening. The safeguard is a specific dose of electricity delivered at a specific time in the cardiac cycle, all synced by the machines. But nothing is perfect. The possible complications mean that we take precautions, but the precautions themselves can fuel trepidation. For a patient to get cardioverted, one of two factors must be established: The patient must have had a TEE (or transesophageal echocardiogram) within the last twelve to twenty-four hours that demonstrates the left atrium is free of clots. Or the patient needs to have been on blood thinners for the past four weeks, at a specific, therapeutic level, verified via a blood test showing that his or her blood is appropriately thin—the INR (international normalized ratio) level—and we have to take the measurement again after more time on blood thinners. If one or both of these preconditions is met, we can proceed. And roughly 90 to 95 percent of cardioversions are successful on the first shock.

After two or more shocks, though, the likelihood of successful rhythm conversion is low; the patient does not transition from AFib (atrial fibrillation) into normal sinus rhythm, and wakes up still in AFib. The danger in successfully cardioverting someone with a blood clot (perhaps in the left atrium) is that changing to normal sinus rhythm may dislodge the clot, pumping it out of the heart. The clot then becomes a loose cannon that can go to the brain and bring on a stroke, or to one of the coronary arteries and cause a heart attack, or to anywhere else in the body, for that matter.

Every time I meet with a patient for a cardioversion consent, I consciously remind myself, the process is not routine. I am preparing someone for what he or she is about to undergo—benefits and risks—and the way I present the information can make all the difference. It's tempting to just gloss over it: "Here's a long list of what-ifs and maybes, but everything's going to be fine, so just sign here. . . ." Tempting, but wrong. Unlike the on-hold recording, "Your call is very important to us . . . ," this *is* very important. It's important information about an important procedure that the patient and family must comprehend. I make an effort to take a highly structured approach, clearly explaining the pluses and minuses: "During this procedure, it is possible, though unlikely, that you could have a stroke and your heart could stop, and, yes, you could die—though, as I said, such outcomes are very uncommon. The benefit of the procedure is that we may be able to make you feel better by putting your heart back into a normal rhythm. Now, if you are comfortable with this, you can sign here. Or you can ask me any questions you might have." The gloss-over-it approach and the deliberate version both constitute informed consent but result in very different degrees of patient comfort. On a personal level, if something went wrong and the patient hadn't been fully prepared, that would be my failure.

My goal is to get each person to understand what's about to occur. Some require more time; some less. Some have questions; some would rather not know. You have to have an inner gauge and give patients what is needed. I don't want to make the procedure seem as safe as getting a haircut, nor do I want patients to feel as if they're about to walk through a minefield. Instead, I aim for balance. Still, this is one of those times in training when a Fellow can feel like an impostor. I'm informing patients of the risks and benefits of a procedure I've rarely seen, and never overseen.

A couple of weeks into the rotation, I'm speaking with a woman in her forties who is, in medical parlance, "scared shitless." Despite the urgings of her cardiologist, she repeatedly put off coming in for her cardioversion. But now that she's here, she dissects every word of the consent. "Wait, what does that mean?" "Hold on. Explain that." "Is that common?" Without the cardioversion, she'll continue to have debilitating palpitations just walking up the stairs in her house. With it, we have a decent chance to make her asymptomatic, or less symptomatic. But she's so obsessed with the risks, it's hard to know if she's going to let us do it. I spend a long time trying to reassure her, using language patients respond to. "While we fully recognize this is not routine for you, we do these every day. . . . We wouldn't have you here unless we thought the chances of your getting better were far greater than the chances of anything bad happening."

If you approach everyone the same way, either too routine or too fear-inducing, you'll strike out half the time. You could say, "When an asteroid hits the earth, only one person in a billion gets hit." And for sure, you're going to get a person who says, "You mean it could happen?!" The challenge is you have about thirty seconds to figure out where to put the patient on the fear spectrum. There are no guidelines based on gender, socioeconomic indicators, clothing, age, nothing. Instead, you need to read the person, his or her facial expressions, understand the reasons behind the tenseness, and act on any clues you can get, fast. It's a challenge, but one that involves responding to people and helping them get the procedure they need. This procedure sounds frightening; all this woman wants is a doctor to recognize and understand her fear, and reassure her. We go through each word of the consent form, point by point. Ultimately, she consents. And fortunately for her (and for her doctors), the procedure is a success.

During week three, one of the attendings I work with is Dr. Richard, a wiry, wired senior faculty member, who does everything in a hurry. He even listens fast, sucking your words up, scanning for key facts, making hurry-up hand gestures so he can cut to the chase and get the problem solved. "Yeah, yeah, okay, let's do it." He's also one of the high-IQ guys who went into electrophysiology because, to him, the arcane web of electrical connections in the heart is a thing of beauty—a Jackson Pollock painting or a schematic of wires and circuits. His passion for electrophysiology doesn't tempt me to consider specializing in this field, but it does give me hope that I'll be as excited as he is about whatever field I choose.

Surprisingly, Dr. Richard has a charisma with his patients that seems at odds with his training and his field. He's all high-speed analysis, data, and deductions . . . until he walks into a patient's room. And then he exhibits a stunning, and frankly surprising, bedside manner. You think he's going to zoom by the patient with his EP-speak—". . . blah-blah-blah, cardioversion, ablation, arrhythmia, catheter, consent. Fine. See you tomorrow"—but he downshifts, taking time, listening, caring. He leads the patient through detailed explanations, answers questions, reducing the most complex technology to layperson's terms. Frankly, I wish he'd slow it down for the Fellows. Patients don't feel dumb asking questions. We do.

Thankfully, there's no such intimidation with the attending for the final week, Dr. Theodore. He was a cardiology Fellow at Hopkins, then an EP Fellow, a nice human being, who does little explanatory sketches. He's methodical and patient, like a high school science teacher. In contrast to some of the others, he makes electrophysiology comprehensible. Seeing patients with him is a primer in translating the arcane to the basic, from Klingon to English, and doing it without being condescending. That's an impressive skill, especially when you're as smart in your field as he is. And he seems to appreciate my input. I generally don't have game-changing EP observations, but he weighs what I say, factors it into the evaluation and decision making. I can't say after the rotation that I'll remember one particular case. But I will remember Dr. Theodore. I want to learn how he makes the jargon of his specialty accessible . . . even if I don't necessarily want to practice in his specific field.

Eventually, even when I get somewhat comfortable with EP, my gut tells me that it's not what I'll do for the rest of my life. Instead, I gain enormous respect for the mental firepower of people who eat, breathe, and sleep electrophysiology. They look at an abnormal heart rhythm like a puzzle to decode, and get very absorbed in it. But I don't find it sufficiently fun. Medicine is not here to amuse me, but as a doctor, I define fun as intellectually stimulating with a human element, and, for me, it's not here. Learning how to get informed consent from a patient was probably the most enjoyable and most useful skill for me. It was the human interaction—rather than the electrical circuitry—that made the deepest educational impression on me.

Still, this rotation becomes a personal reminder that there are some parts of medicine that are so complex, so byzantine, and so abstruse that they're the private domains of the wizards of that discipline. For the rest of us who hope to grasp the big picture of our field, the "whole patient," we aren't going to master the esoterica, nor should we. As a good cardiologist, I need only a rudimentary understanding so that I know when to refer a case to the right subspecialist, just as a primary care physician has to understand when to send a patient to a cardiologist. I suppose the rule is: Know what you know and what you don't know.

10

ROTATION: NUCLEAR MEDICINE, PART II

A Christmas Present

The next rotation is the second round of nuclear. This one, like the first, runs two weeks, which is more than enough for anyone except those who want a career in nuclear stress testing. The first nuclear rotation, I knew almost nothing. I'd never read a scan, and never written a nuclear stress report. This time, I know the drill. As in the first nuclear rotation, I'll read the tests with whichever attending is on, sometimes together, but often not. When we meet, he or she will point out details, comment on my interpretation, add some insight, and ask questions to make sure I get it. No pressure.

Still, I reflexively show up at 8:30 on Monday morning, even though the other Fellows have told me that there's no reason to be there that early. But it's day one, and I'm compulsive. Two idle hours later, I realize the other Fellows were right; there are no scans to read and won't be until they're fed to us by the clinics in the afternoon. The attending isn't here. The door to the nuclear reading room is closed. I drink coffee and read newspapers, have lunch, and return emails. Then, in the afternoon, I go to the lab to meet the attending and get started.

The nuclear reading room is dim, illuminated only by the computer screens surrounding the console where readers—Fellows and attendings—sit in rolling chairs. Today I'm working with Dr. Ulysses, the uncrowned Hopkins king of reading nuclear scans. Dr. Ulysses started in nuclear before the training became formalized, and he has taken every exam and update since. He's also a practicing cardiologist four days a week, not a full-time nuclear reader like some, and to me, that gives him added credibility. In clinic, he sees patients with heart issues, some of whom end up requiring a nuclear stress test. And since he reads scans (maybe not the ones for his own patients but for patients like his), he sees if there is a correlation between the suspected diagnosis and the scans.

When Dr. Ulysses reads the scans, he has an incredible eye for small detail, like an astronomer at a telescope who says, "There's one of Jupiter's moons," but when you look, all you see are fuzzy white dots. Just when you think he's not paying attention, he leans slightly forward, zooms in on one tile, and stares at it with his Superman X-ray vision. He quietly says, "See this?" and honestly, I rarely do. He points to the "before" tile of the same view, then back to the "after," and says, "Right here." Now I see it. His approach as an attending is, he watches you, and if you don't screw up, he just keeps watching. Here and there, he makes a comment: "The anterior wall isn't getting blood." Otherwise, he weighs in only if he thinks you're off. His silence or head nods are his way of giving the okay.

The second day, my attending is Dr. Thomas, who is more intense and obsessive than Dr. Ulysses. She has read scans day in and day out for the past ten years, and will for the rest of her career. She stands behind me, watching me read, and mumbles, "What's that?" I mumble back, "What?" She points: "There, at the septum." She zooms in, "Hmm," then checks another angle. We both stare at the images. She says, "Maybe . . . or maybe not." That's the capsule story of nuclear—and even the experts aren't sure when it comes to reading inconclusive pixels. The images don't shout at you. They whisper, hence the adage that "nuclear medicine" is "unclear medicine." Different attendings look at the same images and draw different conclusions. But the conclusions matter. They help determine whether a patient goes for a more invasive procedure.

I'm not suggesting that doctors should practice without the benefit of technology. Obviously, technology makes the practice of medicine infinitely better, when and if the technology provides a measurable aid. But just as EP attracts electrical engineering geeks, nuclear is a magnet for lab junkies, the ones who love anything technological, and the more complex the better. But sometimes it feels as if we're using technology simply because we possess the tools even when we cannot rely on the findings. To me, this seems starkly different from tests such as cardiac catheterizations that carry clear risks to the patient but also tend to yield unambiguous, actionable results. When I've ordered stress tests in clinic, the tests were attached to people, patient histories, and my own impressions. But nuclear's only setting is the reading room, a room sealed off from the reality of the patients. Maybe divorcing the patient context from the test interpretation makes it more objective, but it strikes me as counterintuitive.

This unreliability of nuclear becomes obvious when the fifth reading falls into the gray area. I think it might be something; Dr. Thomas thinks not. I start to write it up her way, but then she looks again and says, "Actually, there might be something there." We bring in another attending, who agrees with Dr. Thomas's original assessment, so that's what we go with. Somehow, all of this guesswork would be okay if the computer were an arbiter. If a doctor could say "It looks like X" but the computer could counteract with "It's Y," then at least we'd have a fail-safe. But the computer does not diagnose; our subjective, maybe/maybe not readings are the only arbiters. I write up the consensus conclusion and send it to the clinic, where the referring cardiologist now reads our findings, probably trusts them blindly, and acts accordingly. Was there something there or not? I don't know.

Fortunately, in the midst of the nuclear rotation, I also spend time at White Marsh for continuity clinic. This means that, along with the attending, Dr. Andrews, I'm actually seeing real cardiac patients with real problems, and not just scans or photo slices. Funnily enough, one case during continuity clinic ends up altering my view of cardiology because of the tests we do *not* do—a peculiar lesson to learn in the middle of my second nuclear rotation.

My first assessment of Mr. Hawkins is a visual one—a tailored, pinstripe suit on an athletic frame. He wears a perfectly knotted red-and-black tie, silver cuff links, rimless glasses, and his body language clearly says, "I mean business." I take a history, and my first impressions are confirmed: Mr. Hawkins joined the U.S. Navy at twenty-two, rose to a military command position by his early thirties, and retired at thirty-five. He put himself through law school, and now works as a nine-to-five financial planner, and spends his weekends and nights as a volunteer firefighter (his father and grandfather having been firemen). He keeps up with his five kids, jogs a few days a week, and can carry fifty pounds of firefighter's gear into a burning building. As a result, he is in exceptional cardiovascular shape, regularly clocking three-mile runs in eighteen minutes. Eight years and forty pounds after the navy, he's hardly a typical cardiac patient, with no prior heart disease; no hypertension, diabetes, high cholesterol, or tobacco use; and no family history of heart disease.

So why is he here? In order to remain a volunteer firefighter, Mr. Hawkins must undergo routine stress testing at the county health office. During his last test, attached to EKG leads, he lasted fifteen minutes: 50 percent longer than the average forty-three-year-old male, and reported no symptoms. But during peak exercise, his EKG waveforms changed, and seemed potentially indicative of ischemia—arterial blockage of adequate blood supply to the myocardium during heightened physiologic demand.

The question posed by the county administrators is, "Does the wavy line on graph paper mean he has heart disease?" If Mr. Hawkins has ischemia, he's displaying zero clinical indications: no chest pain, nausea, hypotension, or unexpected dyspnea (shortness of breath). As Mr. Hawkins retells his tale, I act as if I'm listening, removing my glasses and putting index finger to temple, even though I know the details from his chart. I'm using the time to think, "What path do we take?"

Do I steer Mr. Hawkins toward the route of least harm or toward a more aggressive one with potential pitfalls? The waveforms in his EKG are abnormal and could be clinical grounds for ordering an advanced test to better define the architecture of his coronary arteries—a cardiac catheterization. But a cath is invasive and carries the risks of bleeding, stroke, heart attack, arrhythmia, and even death. It's not a casual decision. Nonetheless, our system of overregulation, coupled with a fear of litigation, can result in a healthy patient becoming a lab rat. For me, the ultimate gauge is, if the patient suffers complications from tests, whether I can look back and say that ordering them was the right thing to do. If the answer is no, then I don't order the tests.

Every doctor learns the Hippocratic oath in med school, and its implicit maxim, "First, do no harm." It's an unusual vow. Rather than a promise to heal or do good, it's an admonition not to hurt anyone in the name of helping. I decide that sending a robust, symptom-free, firefighting father of three for a cath fails my clinical litmus gauge. I opt to do no harm—or, more accurately, to do the least harm.

But now we come to the crux of the issue: Do we do nothing more? What if that EKG is a clue to something? And what if we send Mr. Hawkins home and he dies of a heart attack that might have been prevented? It can be as challenging to care for the seemingly healthy patient as for the obviously sick because the healthy patient has further to fall. So I take a hybrid approach: I do not order a nuclear stress test, because I don't think it will tell us anything definitive, but I do order an echocardiogram and stress test with ultrasound pictures. The stress echo test isn't perfect. It can produce a false positive or false negative. But it can also provide a measure of diagnostic reassurance without difficult-to-justify risks for a healthy patient. This is one of the greatest challenges of clinical medicine. Since every decision carries risk, it's sometimes unclear which path offers the least harm.

Unlike patients I see during rotations and never see again, I am now involved in treating Mr. Hawkins. When he goes in for the stress echo, as I happen to be in the hospital, I witness the test itself, and not just the written results in his chart. This time Mr. Hawkins is on the treadmill for over seventeen minutes, which borders on the absurd since we rarely expect anyone to go more than ten minutes. And this time, the technician speeds up the track and raises the incline up to a thirty-degree angle. Mr. Hawkins still runs six miles an hour, and even says to the tech, "What else do you want me to do?" Most patients are panting and can't wait to get off, but he's chatting.

The value of pushing somebody is that you can compare the ultrasound pictures taken immediately after exertion to the ones you've taken when the patient was at rest. The longer the patient goes, the more reassured you are by normal-appearing pictures. And it looks as if Mr. Hawkins is fine. He's sweating, but that's normal. And his echo pictures are fine—his heart is functioning perfectly, and every portion of his heart muscle seems to be adequately perfused. We can't see the blood flow, but the normal muscle motion indicates it is adequate. Even though his EKG shows the same quirky wave, in some ways this is actually good, since it indicates that the abnormality isn't a sign of trouble, but is as much a part of him as his bushy eyebrows and oversized feet. In my medical opinion, Mr. Hawkins has had a false-positive EKG.

During Mr. Hawkins's follow-up appointment at the clinic, it's clear that he's doing fine but he's not happy at having been away from his volunteer firefighter's job; it's his way of carrying on the family heritage. If he's okay, he wants to go back right away. That requires an official doctor's letter to give him clearance. And that's a first for me, dictating a formal medical opinion in which I state, for the record, on Hopkins letterhead, that as a member of his medical team, after performing the appropriate tests on Mr. Hawkins, he has a clean bill of health to go back to running into burning buildings. And I, Dr. Daniel Muñoz, MD, have to sign it. Though I imagine this sort of ritual will become routine/commonplace as I progress into my career, right now it feels like a momentous act. I'm officially official.

Sometime later, I wonder how Mr. Hawkins is doing and decide to call his home to check on him. His wife answers the phone: "Doctor, you missed him by five minutes. The firehouse siren always seems to sound when we're sitting down for dinner." That's my answer. All should be well with Mr. Hawkins—at least until the next time the county requires an EKG. Hopefully, the next cardiologist will know that, in Mr. Hawkins's particular case, a restrained approach might very well be the best way to "do no harm." Mr. Hawkins is a case study in the Hippocratic oath, and an important reminder to gather the facts and then trust one's own clinical judgment rather than adhere to a strict algorithmic protocol of testing. Mostly, it's a reminder—again—that we're treating people, not data.

On my last day of nuclear, I'm working with Dr. Ulysses again. We cruise through the reports, and by 7:00 p.m., we're finished. I say, "See you tomorrow." Dr. Ulysses reminds me, "The clinics are closed. Merry Christmas." My two-week rotation on nuclear stress tests was only one week and a day.

Unlike the nuclear testing itself, whose results can be vague (but lucrative), my conclusions about it are clear. The technology behind the tests is impressive; so are some of the practitioners; but the disconnection from patients and the subjectivity of reading outcomes make me question their value, and, as a field, it clearly isn't for me. On the other hand, my midrotation clinic work further reinforces my affinity for direct patient interaction and longitudinal involvement. In fact, by the Sunday after Christmas, my mind shifts to my next immersion. In twelve hours, I'll be back at Hopkins's cardiac intensive care unit. Real patients who are truly sick, and who need constant medical care. I think I'm beginning to know what I like doing.

11

ROTATION: CARDIAC INTENSIVE CARE UNIT, PART II

There's No Such Thing as "Routine"

It's the Monday after Christmas, and I am starting my second rotation of cardiac intensive care, this time at Johns Hopkins Hospital downtown. I will be working through New Year's, which is best described as a hospital's "wacky time," when all the people who somehow staved off every kind of malady to get through Christmas can hold back no more and the onslaught descends. The CICU is packed.

Day one and this rotation is a sharp contrast to the last one. Every bed in the unit is full; every patient is critically ill; several are in heart failure or shock, requiring high-powered IV medications to support their blood pressure. Some patients are contradictions—too young to be so fragile but barely clinging to life, while others are aging miracles, still breathing despite all odds. I've gone from dark rooms filled with computers into the full glare of intensive patient care.

The CICU at Johns Hopkins is a "horseshoe" of glass-walled rooms around the nurses' station, so that the staff can see all the patients at all times. Just like the CICU at Bayview, every one of these cases is presurgical or nonsurgical, ranging from heart attacks, decompensated heart failure, cardiogenic shock (when the heart's pump inefficiency has deteriorated to pump failure), and a variety of dangerous or malignant arrhythmias. Some patients can get out of bed and walk their attachments—a combination of IVs, tubes, wires, monitors, and encumbrances—to the bathroom, or sit up, read the paper, and talk on the phone or to visitors. Other patients lie fully sedated, attached to a mechanical ventilator that breathes for them, while their IVs provide a steady, wide-ranging stream of medications to support their blood pressure. We can monitor all of these patients from the pod in the middle of the horseshoe, on flat screens displaying EKGs, patient names, heart rates, and other vital signs. Audio alarms sound when any patient's readings deviate from the norm (due to anything from an EKG lead that falls off to actual cardiac arrest). All this information is gleaned without stepping into a patient's room, all without human interaction . . . for better or worse.

As with every rotation, there's virtually no orientation or introduction. We get there and do it. My team assembles first thing that morning—the attending, Dr. Chester, a senior professor of cardiology; the Fellow (me); and a team of residents, usually three first-year interns and three junior or senior residents. Together, we'll round on the CICU patients and take care of them day and night for the next two weeks. From 8:00 a.m. until midday, the team moves like a herd down the hall, stands outside each room, and reviews each patient's history and status. There is a highly structured format for presenting a patient anywhere in the hospital—in the ICU, on the general medicine floor, or in obstetrics or pediatrics. It starts with an HPI (history of present illness), one or two rambling, paragraph-long sentences, encompassing all that is meaningful about the patient right now—not all illnesses ever, tangential incidents, or unrelated symptoms . . . and no conclusions yet.

We're here to learn, to teach, and to treat, which takes longer than just treating. The priority is always the patient, not the students or the teachers, but the residents need the chance to learn on their own. Rounding has to strike a delicate balance between the academic side of medicine and proper patient care.

What attendings and Fellows look for are "crisp" presentations, which can be surprisingly hard to define. There are no clear-cut criteria, but a presentation should be short and pithy without omitting anything critical. You can do a good job in ten minutes or a bad job in thirty. An excellent presentation is not unlike what U.S. Supreme Court Justice Potter Stewart said about pornography: You know it when you see it.

The art of rounds lies in the interruptions and the critiques the attendings and Fellows make. A good interruption prompts the resident to expand on a point because it's a salient issue, while cutting in on a presentation and saying "Whoa! You're jumping to conclusions pretty fast" is not only bad form, but incredibly discouraging for a resident. I first learned this on the receiving end, noting that while some Fellows and attendings could deftly interrupt a presentation, others would let the resident wander off course before finally flashing the "T" time-out sign and guiding the resident back to the issue at hand. Hopefully, these experiences will come in handy now that I'm the one doing the interrupting.

The first patient we see is Ms. Jentzen, a sixty-seven-year-old woman who came in two days ago with an ST segment elevation myocardial infarction (MI)—a serious form of heart attack. She had a stent put in, but still needs IV dopamine to maintain her blood pressure. The resident presents the relevant questions of the case: Why is this happening? How long should we continue this course? What's the long-term outlook? It's a good presentation, fifteen minutes, relevant data, and a clear treatment plan, a routine case for the unit. I listen and critique. The attending listens and critiques my critique.

The next patient, a Mr. Orlando, requires a full presentation because he was admitted in the last twenty-four hours. A typical rundown goes through the patient's symptoms, tests, history, other illnesses and conditions, previous visits, medications, family patterns, in order to provide a total physical assessment of the patient. Mr. Orlando also came in with a heart attack, but he is currently sicker than Ms. Jentzen, and thus his case is more complicated.

Dr. Chester, Starbucks grande in her hand, is on one side of the nervous resident who is reviewing the chart. I'm on the other side, peeking at the resident's notes, while two other residents cluster in to learn how to, or how not to, give a presentation. The resident begins, "This is Mr. Orlando, who came in last night with a myocardial infarction because he smokes heavily and is diabetic, has high blood pressure, and was experiencing chest pain." As he goes on, ". . . but he's doing better now. We started him on a beta-blocker . . . ," I know his presentation is heading down a rathole.

I've observed enough of these presentations to know that the most dangerous thing you can do is draw conclusions too fast. If you're a venerated teacher or practitioner, you can do your own version of the format, but if you're a resident, you stick to the book. Or the attending or Fellow will cut you off at the knees. And this resident is doing the unforgivable: He's presuming an accurate diagnosis before getting through the objective data, a critical error. Like a game-show host, the attending, Dr. Chester, zaps him, but her version is a withering scowl: "Doctor, we would prefer to have the facts first and make our assessments afterward."

Then it's my turn. While the attending is a teacher for the entire team, my role is to be a teacher for the residents, and right now, my job is to help the resident without undermining or contradicting the attending. I nudge the resident: "Please review the EKG, the echo, and the enzyme results."

The resident rifles through his papers, which, given the silence, seems to take an eternity. The other residents are collectively holding their breath. Finally, the resident delivers the sequenced facts as he should have—the symptoms, the EKG, the blood work, and so forth—and the attending lets him off the hook, though not without a parting shot of sarcasm: "Thank you. We cannot assume a patient arrived in the ER with a sign over him announcing that he's had a heart attack and that his diabetes and smoking were to blame. The information you've now provided gives us a clearer picture of the situation."

What should have been a ten-minute presentation became a forty-minute case study. But the presenting resident (and the other residents) absorbed the lesson of presenting a spectrum of facts, not presumptions. Truth is the analysis you arrive at . . . if the facts are right.

The conclusion, as expected, is that the patient had a mild heart attack. He's scheduled for a cardiac catheterization to see if further interventions, such as a stent implant or bypass surgery, are warranted. His blood levels are checked to monitor effects his diabetes might have had. In the meantime, he's put on additional heart meds, and his vital signs and blood work will be watched carefully. These conclusions are not dissimilar to those of the resident, but the means by which they are reached are as important as the end.

Afterward, I walk the presenting resident down the hall to commiserate. "We've all been there. Don't worry about it. Nobody died." He nods and thanks me, but I can tell he feels awful.

The attending was rough on him, but she had to be. Her responsibility is to turn residents into good doctors. She doesn't want to send doctors into the world who cut corners or do their job wrong, because a doctor's error can mean a patient's death. Do you tread lightly with students out of sensitivity to feelings, or do you have tough standards that may bruise feelings? Hurt feelings will recover. Patients may not. And Dr. Chester isn't really mean. I've witnessed mean. One attending, after a bad presentation, said to the resident, "Doctor, now that you've leapfrogged over the facts and somehow divined the diagnosis, we can assume this patient is miraculously cured, and we can move on to the next patient so you can perform your magic again. . . ."

But I've also worked with doctors who could skillfully and subtly nudge residents back on track. "So . . . did the patient describe what the chest pain felt like—its intensity, location, duration?" "Can you tell us how the tests did or did not support your observations?"

During the rotation, during rounds, my conscious goal is to emulate and practice that method—"an iron fist in a velvet glove." In addition to the second- and third-year residents, there are interns or first years, and I want to show the younger ones how it's done so they won't have to relearn it later. Out of empathy, I find myself erring on the side of the velvet glove. If residents say something a little off, I raise an eyebrow or try a time-out signal to get them back on script. If the resident says something just plain wrong, I stage-whisper, "Hmm, I don't know." If that doesn't work: "Whoa. Slow down!" The art of interrupting—like being a good doctor—is about knowing when to listen, and when to act.

As week two begins, my interrupting skills are put to the test with three very different residents and a different attending. The attending, Dr. Herbert, has a background in economics and a fascination with technology, and he has a reputation as a fanatic for detail. Many residents, and even some Fellows, find him intimidating. During presentations, he will seize on a hint of incompetence, and he can make even outstanding residents wilt. Nothing annoys him more than lazy doctoring or disorganized thinking. He wants things done right, and he'll grill a resident like a homicide detective if necessary. As a result, some of the residents and Fellows think the right way always means his way. I don't agree. Dr. Herbert is obsessed with advocating for the best care, and has no tolerance for doctors he feels aren't equally obsessed. And when a resident veers off course, Dr. Herbert will bring the process to a halt. He will deconstruct a case for an hour until he's convinced that the resident understands not just that he or she made a mistake, but why and how not to do so in the future.

To get the full, fair picture of Dr. Herbert as a non-ogre, you only have to look at his bulletin board. There are pictures of him, his wife, four kids, and their grandmother, flanked by oversized Berts, Ernies, and Big Bird characters at Busch Gardens or elsewhere on their annual theme park trips. Despite his obsession with medical care, he is very much a human, caring person.

The other evidence of this is that as brutal as Dr. Herbert can be, ripping a resident a new orifice one moment, he can ease a patient's anxiety the next. He can even employ gentle humor, a rare feat in the somber CICU. He's been known to ask, in a very bad French accent, how a patient is enjoying the hospital's "haute cuisine" or to squint at his or her IV tube and say it's time for an oil change. This is the same dedicated but complicated attending who strikes terror in residents, which doesn't always make their work better, but which makes my job of training each of them challenging.

And when it comes to training, there are two basic truths:

1. For residents, at least one patient will get in real trouble in the middle of each night. This is a scientifically proven—albeit baffling—fact.
2. The attending is evaluating all of us—the Fellow, the resident, and the patient. As the Fellow on call, I will be evaluated not only by how the patients fare

but also by how well the residents handle them. It's like treating two people per case.

Every night, I am faced with my end-of-day decision: How long do I stay? Most nights I go home around 7:00 or 8:00 p.m. if I feel comfortable there's a solid plan in place for each patient. But if my pager beeps at 2:00 a.m., I may head back in. There's an adrenalin-like excitement to these moments—a life hangs in the balance—but since I have to return to the hospital at 8:00 a.m., the days can run into one another. Some nights, even before I leave, I know I'll be back. It depends on many things, including the degree to which I feel I can trust the resident on call.

Of the three residents I'm working with, two have good instincts, and can tell when to say "I don't know." Counterintuitively, in medicine, asking for help never makes you look dumb and almost always makes you look wise.

The first resident is a charismatic second-year, a rising-star cardiologist who is so calm, confident, and decisive that he is more or less functioning as the senior resident in the ICU. He's naturally charming, stars in the resident talent skits, and though relatively new to Hopkins, he's become a fixture, the popular kid who is also smart, easy to like, even with a slightly cowboyish nature, meaning he trusts his hunches—right or wrong.

During the evening of his call night, outside the patients' glass-walled rooms, he takes me through each plan. The nurse and attending listen, and his plans seem sound. I'm halfway home when he pages me. A woman in her midseventies, a recent stent recipient, was experiencing worsening hypoxia (oxygen deficiency). He laid out what he intended to do and was calling because he wanted assurance that he was doing it right. He was. It doesn't warrant a U-turn.

The second resident, despite her book smarts—high IQ, very good med school, impressive CV—will rattle off eight different solutions to a single medical problem but be unable to pick one. She's the 800-SAT whiz who can't find her way home from the testing center but carries herself with total confidence because she doesn't know what she doesn't know.

By Wednesday, I am starting to lose patience with young Dr. Book-smart. My concern about her is greater because she is an aspiring cardiologist. This isn't a token cardiac rotation on her way to being a nephrologist or a pulmonologist. And if she's going to be a heart doctor, part of my job is to make sure she's a competent one. The ability not just to glean data but to synthesize it and be decisive is what separates a doctor from a computer. But how do you teach a human Google—all search, no discrimination—how to filter?

On our next case, she begins by giving me all the medical information a doctor could possibly draw upon—GI (gastrointestinal) issues, hematological issues, renal issues—but does not put those issues together. Meanwhile, the patient is in serious trouble, with severe underlying heart failure, bleeding from his gut, and anemia (low blood count). Still, the resident is checking every possible cause and effect, iron studies and B_{12} and folate as possible causes for the anemia. She is wasting everyone's time, including the patient's, by investigating irrelevant vitamin deficiencies and not zeroing in on the real causes.

I try to stick to the "velvet glove" approach. Either I fail or she doesn't get it. I cut in; I ask her pointed questions; I insist on decisions. When she hesitates, I push. I ask her to set out a treatment plan. Finally, I set out the treatment plan and get her to nod in agreement.

Fortunately, the patient responds to the meds and stops bleeding. His blood count goes up a little, which means we can return to worrying about his heart. Still, I go home frustrated with the resident, a little upset with myself for being impatient, and half hoping she'll go into another specialty.

Resident number three is much easier to work with: She's wise, likable, kind, caring, and combines a rosy outlook with competence and a willingness to ask questions. Though she has no intention of going into cardiology (she wants to be an oncologist), she has a good handle on the cases, a calm demeanor, and a way with the patients. I do notice she's a little tentative on the second-to-last patient, Mr. Morton, who is now in the cardiac step-down unit, an intermediate area for patients who are out of immediate danger but are not healthy enough to be transferred to a general inpatient floor/ward. When Mr. Morton first came in, he was in rapid atrial fibrillation—irregular heart rhythm—but since then, he's stabilized, and is on medication that controls his heart rate. I can see that his on-the-cusp condition is making her uneasy, but this uncertainty—and the connection to the patient that it implies—is a good kind of uneasiness for a doctor. It keeps you sharp and attentive, not complacent. We see one more patient before the end of rounds, and, all things considered, I feel pretty good about her assumption of the on-call responsibilities.

The only sleep I've had in the past two days has been a series of nonsequential naps, on sofas and chairs in the Fellows' lounge. I decide to go home and fall sound asleep, but am awakened when the resident who knows enough to ask questions pages me at 3:30 a.m. Mr. Morton, the patient she was uneasy about, has flipped from his steady, slow rhythm into a very fast rhythm. "It looks like rapid atrial fibrillation again," she says. (Rapid AFib can be serious for certain patients, particularly those who are older and/or who have underlying heart disease. It occurs when electrical short circuiting in the top chambers of the heart triggers an abnormally fast heart rate. The heart goes into overdrive— a rapid ventricular response—which can be unsustainable in certain cases.)

I ask, "What's his heart rate?"

"About 160."

"Blood pressure?"

"We're trying to get it. It's like sixty over palp." This is serious. *Palp* means that the bottom number, the diastolic pressure, is so low the machine has difficulty even measuring it.

"Is he awake at all? What's his neurologic status?"

"He's groaning and not making sense." She's trying to be composed and process her steps. Mr. Morton has a completely unstable heart rate, and he's groaning, almost babbling, because his blood pressure is so low his brain isn't getting enough blood flow. She starts to say, "Dr. Muñoz, do you think I should—" but I cut in: "I want you to put the phone down and shock him right now. He's in an unstable rhythm. Shock him with two hundred joules. Now." She says, "Okay." I add, "Page me or call me as soon as you're done. I'm on my way."

I'm almost to the hospital when she pages me to say, "We shocked him; his heart rate is seventy; he's got a good blood pressure. He's annoyed because he hurts from us shocking him, but he's awake and talking." The patient is stable again. The resident knew when to call, and she knew what to ask. Though I had to direct things over the phone, I had a good partner on the other end. Her ability to sort and relay accurate information helped me make the correct management call, and possibly save a patient's life. She knew what to do but just needed confirmation. That's the way it should work.

And then, just when I start to feel as if I have a good grasp on this rotation, a case comes along that flips all the lessons upside down, turns good medicine inside out, and screws up the predicted outcomes.

Stella, age fifty-nine, has an unfortunate combination of high blood pressure, diabetes, bad cholesterol, and obesity. Stella is also a widow, her husband having passed away two years ago, and mixed in with her other symptoms, she shows some residual grief and depression. Depression is a wild card; you never know how it can affect a patient. And then there's her weight. She's under five foot five and weighs 285 pounds. We say that patients such as Stella are "older than their age," a euphemism to soften the reality that Stella is even unhealthier than she looks.

Her diabetes has eaten away at her peripheral blood vessels, resulting in a loss of circulation in (and amputations of) her toes. Stella has what doctors call a "trifecta" of risk factors: (1) diabetes, (2) high cholesterol, and (3) sugar or high blood pressure. Her comorbidities—that is, her other diseases—are conspiring to erode previously healthy blood vessels all over her body. While a toe infection is what brought her to her local hospital, once there she began to experience episodic chest pains, which are much more alarming than her necrotic toes.

The medical team at the outside hospital hooked her up to an EKG, which showed several potential abnormalities that raised concerns about ischemia (portions of the heart muscle not getting enough blood), but not necessarily a heart attack. Stella has signs of unstable angina, chest pain that is unpredictable, and not related solely to exertion. After a day or so without improvement at the community hospital, her doctors move her to Hopkins.

During her ambulance ride to Baltimore City, Stella developed increased chest pressure and diaphoresis (sweating) as well as nausea. The EKG en route indicated ischemic changes (abnormal changes to the electrical pattern of the heart's contraction) that correlated with her symptoms. The good news is that by the time Stella arrived at Hopkins forty-five minutes later, things had calmed on her EKG and she was temporarily symptom-free. However, given her chest pain and our concern for an unstable coronary syndrome, she can't go directly to the vascular surgeons for her toe removal—she has to get "cardiac clearance" before anyone can operate on her.

The first thing that strikes me when I see Stella just before 11:00 p.m. is that she doesn't seem afraid. She's just exhausted, frustrated, and near tears. On quick examination, it's clear that another toe must be removed. Even with antibiotics, the toe is bright red, ugly, and ulcerated. As sick as she is, and as many times as she has been through these amputations, she finds it hard to deal with the loss of another toe.

The first three minutes with a patient are crucial in forming a picture of a case. Observation, visual clues, and nonverbal signals often yield more valuable clinical information than pointed questions. I ask Stella about her chest pain and other symptoms because I'm trying to arrive at decisions on tests, what to do right away, and what can wait until morning. Through it all, she tells me she doesn't want to lose another toe. Privately, I think, "That's the least of your problems," and instead, I try to shift her attention to what's critical. I want to interrupt, "Your heart is the issue tonight," but I also don't want her to panic.

At the moment, since she's not having chest symptoms, we put Stella on cardioprotective medicine overnight and plan for a cath with coronary angiography—X rays of the coronary arteries with dye shot through to illuminate them—for the morning.

Stella gets through the night, and the next day is a Saturday. I don't have to look at a calendar; it's because the rest of the hospital is so quiet. When you're in the ICU, you can't necessarily tell what day or even what time it is. The sense of time or day you do get comes when you walk down a hall into the non-ICU world. Suits and ties—weekday. Short sleeves—Friday and weekends. Empty corridors—late night. Quiet—Saturday or Sunday.

After Stella is taken to the cath lab, the cath team calls me and my CICU attending to show us what they found: coronary disease with one particularly tight-looking, critical stenosis (narrowing) in her right coronary artery. It's a discrete lesion, meaning you can see where it begins and ends. The only blood flow running past it is a thread in a focal section that's fairly proximal—that is, upstream—in the vessel. With

Stella still on the table, we agree the only course is to implant a stent to hold the artery lesion open, hopefully solving her angina issues and clearing one hurdle to her going to the operating room for her toe-related issues.

At this point, we have to decide which type of stent to use. Ideally, we'd opt for a drug-coated or drug-eluting stent, a DES, versus a bare metal stent because the DES tends to remain open longer. That means there's a lower likelihood of scar tissue forming inside the stent, since scar tissue formation can lead to a narrowing of the artery over time. But with the DES, for a full year, patients have to be on both aspirin and the drug clopidogrel, which together act as platelet inhibitors that help blood flow better and prevent clotting. Bottom line: If you're just getting a stent, it's better to get a DES. If there's planned surgery in your future and you can't risk excessive bleeding, it's better to use bare metal and be on the aspirin-clopidogrel combo for one month (as opposed to one year), with only a daily aspirin required after the first month. Stella, who will need to have her toe removed, is getting bare metal.

The stent goes in and I leave to see other patients in the CICU. The cath team pulls out the catheters from her groin vessels, and twenty minutes later, Stella is back in her room, with the nursing staff reconnecting her to various devices. Five minutes later, a nurse tracks me down and says, "I can't get a blood pressure on her." Stella's blood pressure is so low that we can't get a reading at all. In the room, Stella is conscious but ghostly pale. Her heart rate is about one hundred, much higher than when I left her in the cath lab. But her blood pressure is now reading sixty over thirty: dangerously low. I try to ask about other symptoms, but she keeps moaning, "My back hurts. . . ."

With her pressure that low, she could develop a clot that might block off the stent, causing a bigger heart attack. But despite the low blood pressure, Stella is not that tachycardic—that is, her heart rate is fast but not alarmingly so. She could be (a) bleeding as a result of the cath, but also (b) having a "vagal response." When a patient is in a lot of pain from a cath procedure, and/or gets moved in an uncomfortable way, he or she may experience a vasovagal response akin to fainting and losing blood pressure. We give Stella IV atropine to try to reverse a possible vagal response, but it does nothing.

And so far, we've had no luck in changing her blood pressure, which indicates Stella might have a rapid onset internal bleed. If so, that could lead to the leg compartment swelling, the result of hematoma (large blood mass) somewhere along the catheter's path inside Stella's body. Normally, hematomas are easy to spot, but Stella has a great deal of fat around her groin area, making it tough to determine.

There's also a distinct possibility that Stella may have one of the most feared complications, a bleed we cannot see from the outside—a bleed into her retroperitoneum, or the rear area of the abdomen. This would explain her back pain, because an RP bleed can be extremely uncomfortable. And its damage can be far worse than a bleed into the leg simply because you can't see it. Stella has just had needles in her groin for her catheterization, and her weight probably necessitated several attempts to find her artery. Any one of those needles could have sheared or nicked blood vessels and caused an RP bleed. To make matters worse, the RP is a very inaccessible part of the body. It's harder to stop a leak you can't see or easily reach.

There's no time for head-scratching and theorizing. We call the blood bank and tell them that we have a patient with major, ongoing blood loss and that we'll need a continuous supply of blood until her situation changes. The only thing we can do is try to keep up with her blood loss—transfusing blood and pouring fluids into her until the bleed stops. The attending grabs a gown and jams an enormous IV into Stella's leg to get the fluid in now. There is almost no conversation. This is not a teaching moment. Stella's condition is far too critical.

As soon as we get an initial bolus (a rapid infusion or surge) of fluid and blood into her, Stella's blood pressure goes up, her heart rate goes down, and her color comes back. The moment we try to lower the rate of the continuous infusion, her vital signs deteriorate. What we're putting in is just barely keeping her even with what's leaking out of her.

Stella is, right now, our sickest patient in the CICU. She has the full attention of the residents, me, the attending, and the nurses, plural. One-to-one nursing isn't enough. At any moment, there are eight to ten things that need to be done. Doctors are issuing orders, asking for readings, directing traffic, with the nurses in a strategic formation, each performing a task.

We are all focused on getting Stella's blood pressure back to normal, and getting it to stay there so that her organs, including her brain, are perfused. The root cause is, for the moment, a secondary concern. We have to stabilize her before we can fix her—resuscitate her first, then figure out how to stop the internal bleeding. And we have to confirm she really is having the kind of bleeding we suspect before we can try to stop it.

We alert the vascular surgery team, because a bleed of this type and severity cannot be dealt with in the cath lab or the CICU, and it cannot wait until tomorrow. When a pipe bursts, you can shut off the water, then open up the ceiling or the floor, and replace the pipe or cap it off. But the human body requires a constant blood flow—which means that a surgeon has to open the body even while the blood is pouring out.

We get ready to roll Stella's bed to the CT scanner in the basement of the hospital to get a noncontrast (no-dye) scan of the abdomen—to determine if there's blood in the retroperitoneum. Given her instability, there's a chance that Stella will "code," that she'll arrest, and we'll have to do CPR on the spot. We take everything we need with us: the drug box and accoutrements for lifesaving, so I'm ready to run the code, should it occur. Even the ride down is a challenge. We have a woman teetering on the edge of death, rushing to the OR, but to get there, we have to fit all of us and Stella and virtually her whole room—devices, tubes, monitors—into an elevator made for a different era. We roll the bed inside the antiquated box and hit the rear wall, then suck in our guts as the door tries to close but buzzes because the IV pole is sticking out. I tilt it backward and punch the Close button again. The door buzzes a second time, snagging the drawstring of one of the resident's gowns, but finally shuts. Now we just have to hope we don't get stuck between floors. This slapstick routine would be funny if Stella's situation weren't so dire.

Once we get downstairs, the next step is to move Stella onto the CT scan table—while she is still tethered to her devices. We're performing a medical oxymoron, "hurrying carefully": We're in a rush to get the scan but can't afford collateral damage, a dislodged IV, a line pulled out, or an open port. The transfer, from stretcher to body tray, is like passing a full bowl of boiling soup where the bowl weighs close to three hundred pounds and the soup is life support. Six of us—first-year resident, two nurses, two radiology techs, and me—move Stella, three pushing and three pulling. When we get her halfway onto the table, I see a line get taut, hung up in her gown. I say, "Hold on," and everybody freezes, her body in midair, while a nurse frees the line. We start moving her again. The whole drill is so counterintuitive: You have to fight the urge to hurry in order to process and check every part, every sign, to make sure nothing goes wrong.

Finally, we get Stella onto the CT scan table and recheck all connections. Every few seconds, I glance at her blood pressure and see that, in spite of the two units of blood, plus medicine to artificially prop up her blood pressure, she's hypotensive. That is, her blood pressure is heading downhill. I tell one of the nurses to get supporting blood pressure meds from the backup bag I prepared in the CICU, just in case. "Just in case" is happening. We plug in the backup bag. The meds are probably the only thing keeping Stella from arresting and dying.

At last, Stella is ready for the scan. We tilt the monitors toward the control rooms behind the glass shield where we watch the results.

Usually, it's challenging for a nonradiologist to follow the

CT scan, images flashing on a computer screen in real time as the body passes through the scanner. Unless you do it for a living, spotting an abnormality takes a trained eye. This time it's glaringly obvious. There are massive quantities of blood in Stella's retroperitoneum. She has a volley ball–size mass of blood on her right side. It is, unfortunately, what we suspected.

Next step: Get her out of the CT scanner and back on the bed, which is as potentially disastrous as the first transfer. I phone the CICU, giving my attending the update—massive RP bleed, need the vascular team involved pronto—while I focus through the glass on the team moving her back onto the stretcher. The attending tells me the blood bank called to say they've got two more units of blood, and he and I decide to have them ready to hang once we return to the CICU, about three minutes, elevators willing. We cram in, get the doors closed after the usual buzzing, reach the fifth floor again, resituate Stella in the CICU, and continue to infuse her with fluids to support her blood pressure.

The vascular surgery team shows up just as Stella's son and daughter-in-law arrive. They're visibly distressed at the news of Stella's deterioration. The attending intercepts them for an update while I manage things at the bedside. He explains the situation to the young couple—an unenviable task, given that they thought their mom's condition was serious but not life-threatening. Now she's clinging to life. How did this happen? We can tell the family why the cath made sense and what it showed, but we cannot explain why Stella was one of the unlucky few to experience a catastrophic complication.

Inside the unit, the vascular surgeons look at the CT scan

and Stella, and immediately label the case level 1A, the highest rank of emergency surgery. (Level 1 is the highest, but on rare occasions it goes to level 1A.) In terms of the OR, not only does it make the patient next in line, but it renders everyone else—apart from the patients already on the operating table—a secondary concern.

In minutes, Stella is in the OR. The surgeons are not going into the retroperitoneum to evacuate the blood; they're going to the source. They open her leg at the groin level, find the culprit vessel, clip it, stop the bleeding, reattach it, and get out. For somebody this sick, the longer you keep her in the operating room on anesthetics, with an open wound, the worse she's likely to get. The plan is simple: Stop the leak, get out, and hope she's able to tolerate the stress and heal from this life-threatening event.

About an hour after shuttling off to the OR, Stella is back in the cardiac intensive care unit but far from out of the woods. Presumably, the bleeding has stopped, and she's a little more stable. Whether she'll remain that way is the question. Getting a massive inflow of blood and fluids is an unnatural occurrence; when you replace somebody's blood in great volumes, there are a lot of things that need to be replaced along with the blood. We watch and wait and pour electrolytes and clotting factors into Stella as fast as we can.

A side effect of an influx of fluids is enormous swelling throughout the body. This unfortunately causes the pressure in Stella's abdominal compartments to climb to dangerous levels, so high it begins to impede vital blood flow to the tissues in the abdomen. We measure bladder pressure through a catheter, which is a surrogate estimate for intra-abdominal pressure. Normal is fifteen or less. Above twenty-five is abnormal. Hers is over thirty. Those abdominal organs are going to start dying from blood/oxygen deprivation unless we can get the swelling relieved. Unfortunately for Stella, that means back to the OR with the general surgery team.

Thirty-six hours into her nightmare, Stella is on the table, an incision down her abdomen, propped open to provide an outlet for the pressure that has built up. She's now in the SICU, the surgical intensive care unit (one of the few places in the hospital she hasn't been), where the surgeons put on a dressing to cover what would otherwise be her open abdomen. To add to her ignominies, she's intubated, on a ventilator. Twelve hours later—after all kinds of electrolyte abnormalities and acid-based problems—for the first time in forty-eight hours, Stella appears stable. This victory is relative, since it only means that she's not getting worse before our eyes. But there is a glimmer of hope that she might survive.

During the next few days in the surgical ICU, Stella develops what looks to be an acute lung injury from being on the ventilator. The lung problem requires heavier amounts of oxygen through the ventilator, which results in her pulmonary pressure rising to dangerously high levels.

For the moment, Stella is marginally better in terms of her lungs, but her abdomen is still a gaping chasm and the outlook is grim. But each consequent catastrophe has brought her family a step closer to the realities that she, and they, face. In the SICU, the surgical team presents the facts. They're not pessimists, because their nature is to "do," not watch or wait, but they also deal in reality. This is how it is. This is what can be done. This is how it's likely to turn out. Stella's son says, "She wouldn't want this, hooked up to all kinds of things. I know my mother, and this is not how she'd want to live." They've had a few days to witness and process Stella's steady decline, and they're suffering with her. Her daughter-in-law says, "Let's just focus on making her comfortable."

Inevitably, the idea of withdrawing care arises. At first, it's a hypothetical, but gradually it becomes a viable option, then a preferable one. Some people think doctors play God. More often it's the relatives of the patient who make the final call. The ending may be inescapable but the how and when are in the hands of Stella's family. Once they absorb the shock of the impending loss, they have conversations with doctors, with each other, and by phone with relatives who can't be there. In the end, Stella's family decides to withdraw care, opting for "comfort care," which will hopefully make Stella's passing painless and peaceful. A few hours after their decision, she's gone.

Although Stella's family seems to have found peace in their own way, personally I can't shake this case. I've seen death. But I'd never seen a decline this drastic in a patient under my care. A diabetic in the hospital for a routine toe amputation had a precautionary, yet necessary catheterization. Then her blood pressure dropped, and an unexpected internal bleed led to an infusion of fluids, a CT scan, vascular surgery, intubation, and lung complications. . . . The body is not a collection of parts; it's a collaboration that we don't entirely understand. When something major or cataclysmic happens to one part of the body, we can expect other parts to falter—a domino effect.

But that still doesn't fully explain what happened. Or

make it okay. Stella's case sticks with me for weeks, a kind of macabre poster child for when everything goes wrong—and quickly. Even in the structured setting of making the right assessments and the right decisions, death is always a possibility. But Stella's case impresses me with the gravity of what would seem to be everyday medical procedures. There is no such thing as a routine test or even a routine decision. Now every time I order any test or procedure for a patient, I take a moment to envision the worst-case scenario. What if this patient has the most serious complications imaginable? Will I be able to look back and say that ordering the test was still the right thing to do? If the answer is no, I have no business ordering the procedure. In Stella's case, the answer was and still is yes. She needed a catheterization, and faced with the same circumstance, we'd send her to cath again. But now, and perhaps forever, whenever I see a patient, I am reminded of the importance, before I order anything, of asking, "What if . . . ?"

12

ROTATION: HEART FAILURE AND HEART TRANSPLANTATION, PART II

As a Sort-of Veteran

From now until early February, I have my second rotation of heart failure, but this time I'm not as awestruck. It's a cold morning in the dead of winter, but somehow the short days and dark skies lend an appropriate gravity to what I'll be a part of over the next two weeks: determining who's eligible for new hearts, trying to delay or even reverse death sentences, ironically by installing organs from the dying to keep the recipients living—trading one life for another.

On my drive to Hopkins downtown, I think back to my first heart failure rotation and my concern about the "grayness" of the ethical dilemmas involved. What keeps us from dwelling on the "should we or shouldn't we" issue is that most of the time, we can't. There are only a few dozen transplants a year at Hopkins, which means that a lot of people on the list will not get a new heart. Most patients will be treated some other way. The unlucky ones simply won't survive.

The mental tug-of-war starts when somebody does get on the list. As Fellows, we are being trained to do what we can to heal the patient. But what does "healing" really mean? Keeping the patient alive? Guaranteeing a certain quality of life? Should we aim for a better quality of life for a short period or accept a lesser quality because it might mean living for longer? There is no single, conclusive metric we can rely on.

By the time I get to the hospital, my mind-set is back in full heart failure mode. Having looked at the previous Fellow's patient list, I'm ready to make rounds, to see the three patient types: the nos (those who don't qualify for the "new heart list"), the yeses (those who are on the list or will soon make it onto the list), and the vets (those who've gotten a heart and are back for a checkup and/or problem).

I confer with the attending, Dr. Dwight. Only in his midforties—young for a senior heart failure attending—Dr. Dwight is soft-spoken, calm, unflappable yet fully engaged. He doesn't have a powerful presence. Instead, he's a wise and gentle teacher. He gives me autonomy, but I can sense he's paying attention to everything that I do.

One of the things I notice as we go through rotations is that Dr. Dwight is never excitable or celebratory about a transplant. He accepts that, even in successful cases, the patient is likely to have problems, that he or she will still struggle through life. He knows that the reality is not as simple as getting a brand-new heart and a brand-new carefree life to match. He's a realist. I see seven or eight patients a day, and

Dr. Dwight's style reinforces a steady, been there, done that rhythm to my rounds. His affect seems to constantly convey, "Nothing is happening that in some way I haven't seen before." Personally, I have not yet attained that perspective.

Medicine often does a good job of natural casting. If there's a time you want a hotshot—all adrenaline and guts—who believes he can do anything, it's when an ambulance delivers an almost-flatline patient to the ER, or when you send a patient to the OR for a lifesaving operation. As a Fellow, it's sort of exhilarating to be around that kind of cowboy. But for the long-term well-being of the patients, once the heroics are over, they don't need high fives; they need wisdom and care. That's Dr. Dwight.

Toward the end of my first week, a forty-two-year-old man named Cliff shows up. He's a high school history teacher in southern Delaware who received a new heart three years ago—in other words, a vet. If it weren't for his chart, though, I'd never have guessed he'd had a transplant. He's not only a history teacher but a basketball coach, and he's still fit enough to play one-on-one with his kids. But according to Cliff's charts, when he suddenly began having chest pain on a winter night three years ago, EKG and blood tests revealed that he was in the throes of a heart attack so massive that it would have floored anyone in subpar shape. He was put on a breathing machine and hooked up to every kind of life-support medicine, then shipped to Hopkins. The heart attack was so cataclysmic that Cliff was unable to come off life support, because he had barely enough heart cells to keep him alive. And it all came without warning to a nonsmoker with a good diet, no previous heart attack, no prior evidence of cardiovascular disease (other than family genes—father and uncle had had middle-aged heart attacks). To get him off life support, Cliff had gotten an LVAD, or left ventricular assist device, an implanted pump that bypasses the squeezing chamber of the heart and reinserts into the aorta to provide a temporary engine.

While an LVAD can be put in as a temporary solution for a patient waiting for a transplant, in Cliff's case it was put in as essentially the only solution to save his life in the immediate term. There was no way of telling whether a transplant would be an option. A patient can walk out of the hospital with an LVAD, but it's an imperfect solution since it has a driveline that comes out of the body to connect to an exterior battery pack. After a few months, Cliff's driveline got infected. He came in, was treated with antibiotics, had the pus drained, went home, got infected again, came back, was treated again. Because Cliff's driveline was supplying the electricity needed to run the LVAD and his heart, there was no way to take it out, clean the entry point, even find another entry, and put in a new line. Removing the driveline and LVAD would likely kill him. Meantime, the infection was winning, and if Cliff didn't get a new heart soon, it would eventually kill him. Fortunately, after three months on the list, Cliff received a transplant, and had been doing well . . . until now.

Like a good coach, Cliff has played by the rules since he got a new heart. He has taken his meds and stuck to his diet. To keep his immune system in check, he has also followed his immunosuppressive regimen, which unfortunately leaves him more susceptible to infection. He came in for his scheduled heart biopsies, routine visits to look for any microscopic evidence of rejection.

Still, a few weeks ago, Cliff was hospitalized in his hometown with diarrhea, nausea, and general gastrointestinal upset. Ordinarily, patients with diarrhea and dehydration would be sent to bed, told to call in sick to work, load up on liquids, and rest until it's over, but the threshold for caution is lower in transplant patients, primarily because they're on an immunosuppressive regimen. As a result, they're vulnerable. They're taught to be proactive and to report their symptoms early. And doctors are inclined to send them to the hospital. Better to bring such patients in and ultimately find nothing than to not bring them in and miss something important.

With only GI symptoms, Cliff would have been on a regular floor—ordinary problems indicate ordinary treatment. In fact, they teach you early in med school: "When you hear hoofbeats, look for horses, not zebras." Look for the obvious or ordinary and treat it as such. But given Cliff's cardiac history, the situation actually requires a check for zebras, for something out of the ordinary. During my examination, Cliff mentions that his stomach has been bothering him; the diarrhea and a light fever are making him feel "kinda punky." Cliff says, "Doc, I don't know if I have to be here, but I figured I'd tell you guys about these symptoms."

Based on his blood tests and abdominal imaging studies, I'm inclined to agree that this is probably just a garden-variety stomach bug. I confer with Dr. Dwight, who agrees with my take and treatment plan. After Cliff has spent a couple of days in the hospital, we've rehydrated him; he's keeping food down and is feeling a little better. We send blood to the lab to check for the presence of certain viruses, ones that most people could carry without even minor symptoms but that, in an immunosuppressed patient, can wreak havoc. The specific virus we're hunting is CMV, or cytomegalovirus, because in the right host, it can cause systemic (generalized) and organ-specific illness—pneumonia, gastritis, colitis. We check for the presence of viral copies (the number or concentration of a particular virus within the blood). We send a sample of blood to the lab, and the technicians try, through DNA replication techniques, to grow CMV. The results come back: Cliff's blood CMV-PCR (polymerase chain reaction) is negative. And, importantly, his symptoms are improving.

Despite our ingrained caution, this case appears to be a plain old stomach bug. After two more days of keeping his meals down, Cliff says, "I want to get out of here. Sorry to have taken your time." We reassure him that this was the right thing to do. Dr. Dwight and I send him home with a caveat: "If you're not completely better in the next few days, come back."

During the second week of the rotation, Cliff calls to tell us that his symptoms have reappeared. We know how reluctant Cliff is to return to the hospital, so this problem is real. I suggest that it might be time to do a colonoscopy, and Dr. Dwight nods. There are conditions that can hide in the colon—CMV being one—that can infect it without being detectable in the bloodstream. We hadn't kept on pursuing CMV before because Cliff had shown signs of getting better. Now that he's sick again (or still sick), it's time to be sure.

I call the GI team and say, "We've got a transplant patient, and we want a colonoscopy—concern for possible CMV colitis. Can you do him tomorrow?" The GI team agrees. Prior to the procedure, I tell Cliff to hydrate at home. If the endoscopy schedule had been jammed, we'd have kept Cliff home longer.

We have Cliff get prepped for a colonoscopy, which means drinking a gallon of fluid ironically named "GoLYTELY." The "go" part is accurate; the "lightly" part is advertising. It's supposedly flavored—ginger ale or lime or cherry—but the truth is, it reportedly tastes awful. Crucially, it cleans out the colon so that the GI docs can have a clearer view and take biopsies if necessary in their hunt for CMV.

Cliff's treatment team now consists of me; Dr. Dwight; an attending-level gastroenterologist for the procedure; and because of the nature of CMV colitis, Dr. Williams, an attending who specializes in infectious diseases. Dr. Williams tends to recommend an IV formulation of an antiviral medicine, valganciclovir, which will hypertarget the CMV. But dosing it is tricky—it needs to be tailored precisely to the patient's age, weight, and kidney function.

The GI team does the colonoscopy, and, sure enough, Cliff has erythematous (reddened and irritated) patches on the inner lining of his colon. The GI docs biopsy the areas and have them stained for CMV, among other potential culprits. Results usually take twenty-four hours, but we want to know sooner. I contact a colleague over in the pathology lab, and he confirms the preliminary results that Cliff's biopsies tested positive for CMV. And this time, when we repeat the blood work, the CMV shows up there too.

Although CMV isn't immediately life-threatening, the patient's substantial discomfort means that the sooner we can start the IV treatment, the sooner Cliff can begin to feel better.

On Monday, we put in a PICC line, or peripherally inserted central catheter, which goes in like a regular IV but snakes into a deep vessel, feeding medicine to Cliff's superior vena cava. While a standard hospital IV can fall out and lasts about three days maximum, the PICC line is a longer-term IV that a patient can go home with. It also permits administration of powerful medications into bigger, central blood vessels—medications that can be caustic to smaller, peripheral blood vessels that regular IVs go into.

Before Cliff leaves, a nurse walks him and his wife through the home-care routine for the valganciclovir. He'll need to take it once a day in a half-hour infusion. The other twenty-three and a half hours of the day, he'll be comfortable and at home, where there's less chance of picking up some other infection. And a visiting nurse will come to Cliff's home several times per week to make sure he's doing it right.

In the same way that it's difficult to definitively identify CMV, it can be hard to definitively figure out when it's gone. Cliff's symptoms should get better within six or seven days of starting treatment. To assure that the infection doesn't recur, he will need to come back to the transplant infectious disease clinic and the heart failure clinic over the next few weeks. I keep tabs on him through the electronic medical records, and conversation, and it seems that he's doing better. But Cliff will always be a transplant patient, always vulnerable, with doctors who are appropriately paranoid, looking for the next threat.

Cliff is a perfect case in point that the typical heart transplant patient's life, after the initial miracle, isn't dramatic; it's actually dull and monotonous, meticulously monitoring everything, most of which turns out to be nothing, but which could be something. A transplant isn't a cure; it's a stall, a walk through a minefield, slow and tedious, even boring . . . unless something blows up. For Cliff, this time it was CMV. Next time it will be something else—a respiratory infection, a cut that doesn't heal, a urinary infection. The rest of his life, which we hope is a long one, will require a proactive, risk-averse attitude on the part of Cliff and his doctors. Not only will we tolerate hypochondria, we will encourage it. Overreacting is good. Boring is good. It means a longer life.

That Friday, I leave around 6:00 p.m. For heart failure, it's been an instructive but unremarkable day. Cliff went home. And he's immediately replaced by other Cliffs.

An hour later, I'm having sushi when my beeper goes off. It's a message to call a Mr. Mann about his son Richie. Mr. Mann asks, "Is this the heart failure doctor at Hopkins?" I say it is, and he explains that Richie is an outpatient of Dr. James, an attending on the heart failure service. In a very calm voice, Mr. Mann tells me that Richie's defibrillator has gone off eight times in the last hour, as if he were mentioning they had to reboot their computer. I start scribbling information on my place mat. A very young man with an implanted defibrillator (an internal device that delivers electric shocks to the heart to reestablish normal sinus rhythm) is hardly routine. So when Mr. Mann asks, "Is this something we need to worry about?" I'm already thinking

"Worry? How about panic?" but tell him that he should call 911 and/or proceed to the nearest emergency room and that I'll get back to him shortly.

I pull up Richie's record on my computer: late twenties, familial cardiomyopathy. (One of my earlier patients, Malcolm, who was in his thirties, flashes through my mind. This guy is even younger.) There's a family history of heart failure of unknown cause, one of those infamous "idiopathic" cardiomyopathies, the ones that "just happen." Richie's heart function is so poor that he's at constant risk of sudden cardiac death from bad rhythms. The only thing that may save him is pacing or shocks from the defibrillator in his chest. His eight shocks in an hour are at least six more than the average crisis. He needs to get to a hospital, immediately.

Later I learned why his father seemed so unflustered. He himself had been through this same ordeal a couple of years ago and had gotten a heart transplant. In Mr. Mann's case, he'd had a known cardiomyopathy and developed what's called "VT storm." VT storm is a recurrent, refractory—as in not yielding to treatment—ventricular tachycardia that can rapidly degenerate into clinical instability and impending cardiopulmonary arrest. Like his son, Mr. Mann had a defibrillator, and then one night, he went into VT storm and received shock after shock. The defibrillator is programmed to deliver lesser jolts or stimulus, called antitachycardial pacing, or ATP, and only if these don't get the heart into normal rhythm does the defibrillator send out the big shocks. The small shocks aren't too uncomfortable. The big shocks are like getting whacked with a baseball bat in the sternum. The whole body jumps off the table. Again and again. As a result, Mr. Mann thought that a few shocks from a defibrillator were pretty routine, until Richie got up to eight shocks an hour. Only then did he think to call the doctor.

I phone Mr. Mann back: "Have you called an ambulance yet?" I don't want the family to panic, but I make it clear that this can't wait. Don't take a leisurely drive down to Hopkins. Go immediately to the nearest ER. I want Richie on IV anti-arrhythmic medications to try to quiet his heart down. His father may be unflustered, but Richie is flirting with death.

I leave a message about Richie's condition with Dr. James, the essence of which is, if Richie can be stabilized at the local ER, he should then be transferred to Hopkins tonight. Dr. James, who is at his son's basketball game, calls me back and agrees.

By the time I connect by phone with the hospital where Richie is being treated, they're preparing him for transfer. His defibrillator has shocked him twelve more times, and they're loading him with IV amiodarone to try to electrically stabilize his heart. The amiodarone is calming his heart as much as it can, but that isn't much. The ER docs know that their hospital won't be able to do much more for him and nothing good will happen if Richie stays there. They decide to helicopter him to Hopkins to the cardiac ICU. On the half-hour ride, Richie is shocked every few minutes.

This is the first case I've been a part of where a patient is in this much trouble before he even arrives at the cardiac ICU. I want to be there. There will be another Fellow on duty and a resident, both members of the CICU team. But I got the initial call from Mr. Mann, and I want to see this case through. More than anything, I'm curious. I want to see what this looks like.

I arrive a little after Richie does, at 10:30 p.m. He has his IV medicine, but he's still sore and exhausted. For over six hours, his heart tried to stop beating, and each time, a machine whacked him in the chest. His body and his mind have been through hell. And Richie is no weak-looking character. He's bulky, with a mullet hairstyle, facial stubble, and tattoos—the kind of guy you see on a Harley on I-95 and make sure you don't cut off. But he's also kind and soft-spoken when I talk to him in the cardiac ICU (and one tattoo says *Gramma*). He tells me that the real pain isn't in his chest; it's in his right shoulder. The shocks from the defibrillator have reaggravated an old shoulder injury—each time Richie got shocked, he buckled over and clutched his shoulder. He's had this problem in the past, resulting in a partially torn rotator cuff: an extra pain he didn't need.

I explain to Richie that I'm there on behalf of Dr. James, which reassures him. All of a sudden, he gets shocked again. He'd gone into VT while we were talking. Richie lets out a wild "Yeooow!" that ricochets through the unit as his monitors go off. But the jolt puts him back in normal rhythm, and he's "electrically quiet" after that. The nurses reload him with amiodarone, which helps to calm his heart for now.

I grab a little sleep and see Richie the next morning. Dr. James and I talk to the CICU team about his case. There isn't a lot to do. The medicines are doing what they can. The defibrillator is ready to fire. After years of heart problems, Richie now has a baggy, floppy, weak heart with short circuiting that will only get worse. Richie's arrhythmia is due to the progressive, irreversible decline of his heart. There's no way to definitively fix it, at least not with the heart he has.

All we can do with medication is attempt to quiet things

down; the goal, for now, is to buy time. Over the next three days, Richie has a few more VT episodes, more shocks, more bucklings and clutchings. Orthopedists come to look at Richie's shoulder, and fit him for a stabilizing sling so that he can move around in less pain. At the moment, he can just about drag his IV to and from the bathroom. He's considered stable right now, but that only means he's not about to die.

Because of his condition, Richie goes straight to the top of the transplant list. Since Richie has been followed by Dr. James as an outpatient, many of the required steps have been completed, which means we can expedite the rest of the process. Clearly, Richie can't leave the hospital. He can barely get out of bed. All we can do is wait and hope his name comes up soon as a potential recipient of a new heart.

The CICU team checks on Richie throughout the day, as does my group, the heart failure/heart transplant team. The CICU team keeps him alive and stable. My team is there to make sure he remains a good candidate when and if a heart is found. His father visits often too. Some of the nurses remember him from his own transplant. These days, Mr. Mann looks so healthy that his presence lends an irrational optimism to Richie's case.

During the wait, Richie's heart experiences a period of relative quiet. His mother and father wait with him, along with an uncle who also had a heart transplant—there's no denying Richie's genes. His brothers and friends are there around the clock. This was a moment they'd all known might come for the better part of Richie's adult life: the day when he might lie in a cardiac care unit waiting for someone else to die so that he can live. And that day is now.

As it turns out, Richie doesn't have to wait that long for a heart. He has two factors working in his favor: First, his rank is high (a dubious honor given his condition). Second, his blood type is AB positive, which means that Richie is a match with almost any other blood type.

When a member of the CICU team delivers the news to Richie that it looks as if a heart has been found, I'm down the hall with another patient. But when I walk past his room, I see a moment that speaks more than words: Just inside the sliding glass door, Richie's mother sits next to his bed, teary-eyed, holding his hand and stroking his forehead. Just outside of the room, Richie's father is talking to a visitor, outwardly calm, like a veteran whose son is heading off to war. The picture is indelible. It captures fear, hope, and even the difference between mothers and fathers.

A heart's journey can be a story in itself (albeit a fast one, since the donor heart can't be deprived of oxygen for too long). A heart can come from Hopkins's own ER, literally down the hall; or from the Baltimore City Detention Center; or from the scene of a motorcycle accident. There are countless macabre but medically fruitful situations.

Confidentiality is a factor too. Patients are not supposed to know where the heart comes from, or how the donor died. Although patients might be appreciative, they generally can't go find the donor's family and thank them. There's little upside to making a connection between recipient and donor. The doctors may know, but, if so, they keep it to themselves. We try to view the donor as an extension of the organ, and not so much as a person. Otherwise, the emotional and psychological subtleties can be a lot to deal with.

Now that the heart is on its way, medical activity surrounds Richie. Blood is drawn and sent for analysis. Anesthesiologists check him out and explain what they'll be doing. The cardiac surgery and cardiac ICU teams come in. Med students and residents come and go. For the next three hours, while all the prep proceeds, we're aware that the whole event could be called off at any moment, for any number of reasons. New medical information about the donor may come to light; the organ-procuring team may encounter issues with removal; the weather may interfere with the procurement team's ability to travel between the organ site and the hospital; the patient may deteriorate too much, too fast.

The transplant is scheduled for Richie's sixth day in the CICU. An imposing, grown man who, because of his heart condition, has had to live with his parents and cannot get or hold a regular job is about to receive a new heart. This operation could change his life forever, if he survives it.

That afternoon, after all the protocols are met, Richie is wheeled into surgery. The operation will take almost five hours. Whenever I walk past the waiting room, I see his family pacing, drinking coffee, and quietly trying to reassure one another. But for most of that five-hour stretch, I'm in the operating room theater, watching as a team of surgeons performs a riveting—albeit slightly gruesome—ballet. Each surgeon has a highly specific job, and all of their steps are orchestrated precisely. They open Richie up, saw his sternum down the middle, and spread the rib cage to either side.

Then Richie is put on a cardiopulmonary bypass machine, which allows his major arteries and veins to be cannulated (insertion of tubes to divert blood flow), and subsequently drained completely. His blood now runs through the bypass machine, allowing this car-size contraption to act as his heart and lungs during the operation. The size of this machine is its own testament to the power of the human heart. It astounds me that we are born with a fist-size muscle that requires a device that large to stand in for it.

Once Richie is connected to the bypass machine, his own heart is removed. It's a dramatic, frankly solemn, sight. For heart doctors, it is an unforgettable visual justification of all that we do. I spend a moment taking it in.

Next, the donor heart is formally implanted; all the veins and arteries are sewn together, after which they're checked and double-checked by team members. And then, carefully, gingerly, the surgeons detach Richie from the bypass machine. When they make that switch, his new heart is supposed to take over. His blood is supposed to start being pushed through his body, but by someone else's heart. If the heart doesn't start immediately, the only possible recourse is to jolt it electrically. But you can't put the old heart back in. The new heart has to work. Everyone—no matter how many times they've seen it or done it—holds their breath.

With all eyes fixated on the new heart, we wait. There's no switch to turn it on. At this point, we're relying on biology and nature, on the heart's ability to recognize connections and to decide that it's going to start beating again . . . if it's going to. It beats once. That single thump is miraculous to me and, I think, to everyone in that room, no exceptions. My naïve, inexperienced expectation is that the donor heart will now start beating regularly immediately. No. It has to work its way there. After the first beat, there's at least a ten-second pause, which can feel like ten minutes. And then, eventually, a second beat. Slowly, steadily, over the next thirty seconds, the beats become more frequent, more organized, more forceful, more reliable. After what seems like an eternity, this new heart is beating regularly. It has decided to start working again, this time in an entirely different body.

That evening, nearly six hours later, Richie lies in the cardiac surgery ICU. This is a postsurgical ICU, so it's run by the surgeons, and it's all about monitoring the recovery after the physical trauma of having your chest cracked and your heart patched, bypassed, or replaced. Richie has an endotracheal tube down his throat, which, along with all the IVs and monitors around him, gives him a strangely mechanical look. He's still full of anesthetics, and he will likely need a machine to help him breathe for another twenty-four hours, during which time the anesthesiologists will guide him from deep sleep to full consciousness. His family looks in on him, and their relief and anxiety are palpable. You made it, their expressions seem to say. Now wake up, please wake up.

When Richie finally opens his eyes, the breathing tube prevents him from talking. He has a zipper scar up the middle of his torso, a bit longer than a typical bypass scar, and he has drains coming out of him to get rid of any excess fluids and/or detect bleeding. But now he could easily be mistaken for any other patient with a serious heart issue, not the borderline marvel that he is. But unlike other heart patients, he didn't come to Hopkins for a pacemaker implant or a valve replacement or bypass surgery. He came for a new heart, one of only a handful per year. Ten days ago, Richie was barely alive. And now he's in the process of recovering with somebody else's heart. In medical parlance, pretty f—ing amazing.

A few days later, after being freed from the breathing machine and now fully awake, Richie is moved out of the cardiac surgery ICU to Nelson 6, the cardiac surgery general ward. I see him every day, usually twice, on my rounds. His father, the transplant vet, visits him daily, as does his mother. As the days go by, I see Richie's brothers and friends less and less—a sure sign that their confidence in his survival is rising.

One day, his brother catches me in the hall and asks how I think Richie is doing. It's an interesting question. Richie has been battered, beaten, and sliced open, and he's trying to get used to an alien organ. But his condition is nothing short of amazing compared to what might have happened with no transplant—in which case, he'd likely have died in days or weeks. The period of greatest danger is up to and through surgery and immediately following. Some patients don't get off the operating table, but Richie did. Days, weeks, and months later, the outlook becomes measurably better. I give his brother the standard medical answer: "Under the circumstances, just as we would hope at this point."

Right now the prognosis for Richie, or someone in Richie's situation, is "good" with an asterisk. He'll see his clinical cardiologist frequently at first, then four times a year, then twice a year. He'll live on immunosuppressant medications for the rest of his life. He'll invariably have bouts of jeopardy as Cliff had. The asterisk is how we measure "good." Unfortunately, compared to normal male life expectancy, the rest of Richie's life is an actuarial estimate. About 85 to 88 percent of transplant patients live a year or more; 76 to 79 percent live at least three years; 67 to 72 percent live at least five years. And the longevity is improving. Male transplants tend to live longer than females. According to the numbers, Richie has a reasonable chance of long-term survival. As of this writing, the longest-surviving transplant patients include: Tony Huesman (over thirty years, ultimately dying of cancer), John McCarthy (thirty-one years), and Lizzy Craze (thirty-plus years). Kelly Perkins, who survived nineteen years, climbed Mount Kilimanjaro six years after her transplant. Dwight Kroening, a twenty-two-year survivor, finished the Ironman competition. (Dwight's luck also held as he ran the 2013 Boston Marathon but a leg injury kept him from the finish line to miss the bombing.) These patients have all come a long way since Dr. Christiaan Barnard performed the first transplant, in 1967. His patient lived eighteen days, a miracle at the time. Richie's prognosis is good, with an asterisk, but the footnote is changing in his favor.

Two weeks and a day after arriving at Johns Hopkins Hospital, Richie and his new heart were sent home. Richie's case—one of heart failure's "yes" cases—was a medical rarity. It was a learning experience for me, and one I was lucky enough to see all the way through. But for every uplifting case, there are always a few that foment cynicism.

Around the time we're all crossing our fingers for Richie, in walks Zelda. "Zel" is sixty-three and has a long history of cardiac issues. She has smoked for most of her life, and has poorly controlled high blood pressure plus high cholesterol:

the full spectrum of coronary risk factors. No surprise, she's had several heart attacks, each one damaging a little more heart muscle, leaving her with a severe case of congestive heart failure due to coronary artery disease. Even though Zel had a bypass, as well as stents, her heart continued its progressive decline, even with an oxygen tank and lots of meds to keep her going. But Zel managed to quit smoking a few years ago, because she needed a transplant, and not smoking is a cardinal rule: Smokers don't get new hearts, just as drinkers don't get new livers.

Over the next six to nine months, Zel was monitored closely by her cardiologist, referred to Hopkins for a formal transplant evaluation, and put on the transplant list. Like Richie, Zel had a favorable blood type, so the wait wasn't excessive. After she received a new heart, her story appeared to have a happy ending. A patient with bad coronary artery disease and multiple heart attacks, largely due to a self-abusive lifestyle, finds cardiac religion and gets a lifesaving operation.

Not quite.

A lot can go wrong with a transplant, even with a patient who has made significant life changes. The body can reject the heart, develop infection, or die. That's why getting on the list is so selective and so specific. But human nature still throws this process for a loop: We cannot factor in the idea that, with some people, things can go *too* well. If the transplant is a success, the patient feels much better. The symptoms of heart failure—shortness of breath, edema, swelling, abdominal girth, nausea, overall fatigue, inability to lie flat, inability to walk across a room—all tend to go away. And when people feel healthy, they start to think there's nothing wrong with them. They think they're "all better." But they're not. As one of the other Fellows said, "Give some people a new heart and it affects their brain. They get 'cardiac amnesia.'"

And according to what I glean from Zel's chart and computer records, she has developed a very serious case of cardiac amnesia. Bit by bit, she reverted to her old bad behavior. She missed appointments with the transplant team and didn't reschedule them. She was lax about taking her immunosuppressant medication. Amazingly, she even started smoking again. A new heart, with a new set of coronary arteries, tends to develop disease faster than the arteries in the original heart. And that's without smoking. When you throw in a pack of Marlboros a day, coronary artery disease is off and running. And nothing the doctors say seems to deter Zel.

I call Dr. Dwight and say, "We have this lady who's a mess, a transplant six years ago, congestive heart failure, off her meds, no recent biopsies. . . ."

He sighs. "Yeah, I know her."

"What tactics have you tried? What do you think would be helpful?" I ask.

His voice is resigned. "We've tried everything. This is what she does."

Ten years after being diagnosed with heart disease, Zel has gone from a textbook success to a case study in regression. She's still alive six years after her transplant. On paper, her case looks like a testament to Hopkins's quality of care, an outcome that boosts our reputation. But along the way, she has probably consumed millions of dollars in healthcare resources, far beyond what her insurance covers. And worst of all, she has taken someone else's healthy heart, and, whether she sees it this way or not, has flagrantly mistreated it.

To be fair, Zel isn't a mean person. She's tough but sweet, loves her pickup truck, and cracks crude jokes. But it's hard to find her attitude—"What heart condition?"—funny or charming. She treats the hospitals and the doctors like her personal pit crew. When she breaks down, she rolls in and the experts check her vitals, stick tubes in her, take the tubes out, then put her back on the road, so she can do damage to herself all over again. Meanwhile, someone such as Cliff has a heart attack at thirty-nine, takes his meds, exercises, shows up early for his appointments, and may not live as long as Zel due to the inevitable complications that can arise from being chronically immunosuppressed on antirejection medications.

We put Zel on a regular cardiac floor. I examine her. When I listen to her lungs, I hear a crackly sound in the lower lung fields. That's fluid, or pulmonary edema. If you have fluid overload, when you lie flat, it can be uncomfortable and cause a labored breathing noise. Fluid that collects in the body takes the paths of least resistance—to the legs, the soft tissue, the lungs, the belly, wherever it can reside. Zel has it in three or four places. I also look at the veins in her neck. They are visibly bulging, a sign of increased pressure, which means that her congested heart is working too hard. And to make the situation even worse, Zel ran out of her medications two weeks ago—medications designed to keep the fluid abated and her heart from overworking—but she hadn't bothered to refill her prescriptions.

I probe: "How did you run out of medications?" (It's not

hard to count. There are only so many days' worth in a bottle.) She shrugs. "I just did." I persist: "When you were running low, how come you didn't get a refill?" Another shrug. "I just didn't think about it."

With the medicines we have in the hospital, it's relatively easy to get the excess fluid out. We put an IV in and pump her full of diuretics. Right away, Zel starts to feel better because she's dumping liters of excess fluid each day, by urinating it out. It's exiting her legs, her belly, and her lungs. She's not as achy, she's carrying less weight, and she can breathe more fully. She feels better, which is double-edged. For the twentieth or fiftieth or hundredth time, she thinks she's all better. Which means she can go do the things that will send her back here. Of course, she swears this time she gets it. This time she's going to take care of herself. This time . . .

On her last day at Hopkins, I give her a version of the "Life or Death" speech. Though it's likely an exercise in futility, I make my last-ditch effort. Despite all Zel's self-destructive behavior, I want to believe that I can get through to her. "What you're doing to yourself is going to kill you. It's not a matter of if, it's just when," I tell her. "And you have to stop smoking. If you want to live, you'll quit. It's up to you."

Dr. Dwight is less impassioned and more realistic than I am. Patients such as Zel are one of the reasons doctors such as him don't get starry-eyed about transplants. He's seen the good ones and the bad ones. He even empathizes with her: It's human to want to believe you're fixed. It's human to deny reality. Dr. Dwight doesn't condone her attitude. But, as a realist, he knows that this can happen. He, and now I, have witnessed the injustice in the Ms. Zels who seem to have nine, unearned lives while there are people such as Cliff and Richie who cling to theirs.

Dr. Dwight's tempered demeanor befits the field of heart transplantation. And, I realize, maybe mine does not. Transplantation offers hope. But it does not do the impossible. Even when it can overcome human physical flaws, it cannot overcome human nature. For me, I know it would be hard to keep making an emotional investment in people who don't want to invest in themselves. The fear of dying, the chance at a new organ, the screening process itself, may motivate patients to change their bad behavior. But all the fear, all the promise, and all the screening panels and teams of multidisciplinary experts cannot predict when the change is temporary, when the patient will miss appointments, fail to take medication, and take a new heart and a new life for granted. But it's hardly black-and-white; for every Zel who flouts the rules, there's a Cliff who does everything he can to save his own life. My goal is to help people who want help. Maybe I am asking too much.

13

ROTATION: ECHOCARDIOGRAPHY, PART I

Little Pictures in a Quiet, Dark Room

Though the rotation order is random, sometimes the timing works in our favor. My previous high-adrenaline rotation is followed by the technically complex, but otherwise low-key, echocardiography. And the next two weeks lead into my vacation, coming at the end of a calendar year that has been intense. (You don't realize how draining rotations are until they're over and you still feel the impact.)

Echo is decompression. There are no minimum or prescribed requirements. How many echoes you read and how involved you are in the lab depends on you, your personal degree of interest, whether you plan to make this your career or not. You have to be present to help supervise stress tests, and to read some studies each day, but the expectations are largely self-set.

I arrive at 8:30 in the morning, get a double espresso to

stay awake, and head into the echo lab. It's filled with computer screens and operates in relatively real time, meaning the studies are done by technicians at the patient's bedside, or elsewhere in the hospital, or remotely at a clinic, and the images are electronically beamed to our station. The lab is small and windowless, a distinct contrast to dealing directly with real patients in the bright white light of the CICU, or heart transplants, or the outpatient preventive clinic. Going from a bedside with sick patients—worried families, life-and-death situations—to staring at magnified images with a little pointer requires something of an adjustment. The reading is a daytime activity, with routine studies done as they come in, unless bumped by an urgent or emergency study (such as in the medical or cardiac intensive care unit or the emergency room). To me, echo resembles a slow-motion videogame: I read the echoes, then an attending reads them, and the reports become final a few hours after they come in.

Each echo is a picture, or series of pictures, of the heart created by high-frequency sound waves that bounce off solid objects but pass through liquid and soft tissue. Just as with any kind of ultrasound, gel is put on the patient's chest, and then a probe is moved over the area to give several different perspectives. The result is a moving image of the heart and the valves within. It's incredible technology and can reveal a lot: the size of the heart chambers, the thickness of the walls, whether the heart muscle is working properly. But to the uninitiated, an echo is just a series of fuzzy snapshots of pulsating body parts.

The echo attending, Dr. Millard, is a gentle woman in her midforties who reads scans all day. An expert spirited away from a renowned midwestern medical center, Dr. Millard has dedicated her life to echo. She also has what we call "a brevity aversion," meaning that she never answers a question in less than fifteen minutes. My orientation alone takes almost an hour, far more than needed, but a testament to Dr. Millard's being so invested in making this rotation as meaningful as possible.

After the intro, Dr. Millard has me reading studies right away. I go through them one at a time, very slowly. The stakes are low and the pace is regular: We read, we interpret, we report. If I'm unsure, I hit Replay, or adjust the brightness or pixel detail, and rerun it. Whether I take five minutes per study or an hour, it doesn't seem to matter. As the Fellow in the lab, I have time. It's pretty isolating, so I have to leave the echo lab occasionally to talk to someone outside the room, on another floor, or at the coffee shop, or to visit the bathroom to get rid of the coffee, or to go anywhere but the lab to return to planet earth.

On some rotations, the Fellow takes on a good deal of the workload from the attending. Not true in echo. Whatever I read, an attending also reads. I compare what the attending saw with my reading on every study. The final report is the attending's, not mine. I learn by observing how a read by one person becomes a group consensus.

In the beginning, it takes me a full hour to complete each study—to look at all the images from every angle before I can offer a preliminary assessment. That same prelim report that takes me an hour takes an attending six or seven minutes. My first reports are essentially extra work for the attendings, who have to read, comment on, and correct my work in order to lead me to the right observations and interpretations. I try not to interrupt the attendings with too many questions, because their first priority is to plow through the studies and get timely, accurate reports out. I put what I conclude into objective data for the report, plugging it into a template that prevents you from getting too verbose. There's even a Commentary drop-down menu so you don't have to write out "Aortic valve is without stenosis." Instead, you click the "No aortic stenosis" option. Although the automation is handy, it reinforces for me why this rotation is more like a technology app than patient care.

Toward the end of the day, Dr. Millard will usually volunteer input. The attendings on this rotation often make use of the "shit sandwich": compliments on the outside, criticism inside. "Dan, on this echo, you got these aspects [pointing to the images] totally right. I just wanted to talk to you about this aspect [pointing to another image], which I interpret a little differently. . . . Except for that, you did a good job interpreting the study." When I'm wrong, Dr. Millard takes me through the images and instructs me on how to discern and measure, how to see what she sees.

In the middle of week one, I read what appears to be a straightforward result, a measurement called the "ejection fraction." The ejection fraction reflects the efficiency of the squeeze of the left ventricle, and for a healthy heart, a 60 to 65 percent ejection fraction is normal. It can be higher in states of hypercontractility (excessive cardiac wall motion occurring, for example, in a septic or dehydrated patient), or lower in cases of heart failure or after a heart attack, as low as 5 or 10 percent. The estimate of the squeeze of the left ventricle is based on different pictures, different cross sections, and images that show the left ventricle contracting. My prelim report on this particular patient's study is 45 percent. Dr. Millard thinks it's more like 55 to 60 percent. I'm not way off, but I'm off compared to the veteran, which is a useful lesson in why my report is the preliminary one, and an incentive for me to review the images. This is a visual assessment, not done by a device that measures the percentages. There are some quantitative tricks of the trade, but no perfect measure. As long as you're in the same ballpark, it's fine.

It's a stress-free rotation, because even when you're corrected, the focus is on learning. The environment is more collegial and academic than other rotations. However, each review tends to be short, and for good reason. Attendings spend thirty seconds or so on any single clarification because they have to keep pace with sixty or seventy studies a day—a report every seven minutes—and they cannot leave any unread at the end of the day. The bean counters who keep the hospital in black ink would likely come down hard on unread studies.

The volume of studies, and the pressure to get them out quickly, are good medicine. High-quality, timely reports lead to faster, better treatment. But logic says there's an economic factor too. Echo exists primarily to serve Hopkins patients, Hopkins clinics, and Hopkins doctors. However, on certain occasions, we get studies sent from other hospitals; more volume, more pressure, but also more revenue. The number of doctors a hospital maintains to read echoes is a clear sign to referring doctors, patients, and the medical community at large that the hospital is a thriving cardiac center, with commensurate revenue streams. It's simple:

Much of what we do in medicine loses money. Echoes bring in money.

But, when you're the Fellow, a rotation such as echo gives you downtime—that is, time to think. I find myself wondering about cases from past rotations. I go into the EMR (electronic medical record) and look at patients' lab reports. I seek out another Fellow, now on heart failure, and ask how Cliff is doing. I ask another if he's seen Malcolm.

Sometimes I walk over to the CICU if I have a few minutes to see which of the patients I might know. When you go into someone else's rotation territory, you're careful not to intrude, not to offer advice or input, just get an update. We don't know enough about what went on before we saw that patient, and what will come after. We try to extrapolate in snapshots backward and forward, but we don't see the whole picture. In spite of that, we try to make decisions not only about patients but about ourselves and our futures based on these limited exposures: I'm going to be a heart failure doctor because I thrive on the intensity . . . or, rather, the intensity I experienced for my particular four weeks. I'm not going into electrophysiology because EP is technical and detached . . . at least during my few weeks of it. I like continuity clinic. I don't like nuclear. I'm interested in interventional. A monthlong rotation is fellowship's maximum length of time to attempt to focus, concentrate, and minimize interruption. We do care about the patients. We get attached. We root for them. But we don't usually know what happens in the long run. We've gone on to the next rotation. Most doctors in training come to accept it. Some even opt for specialties virtually cut off from direct patient care, such as nuclear or echo, marketable skills but not patient-interactive. That works for some doctors, but not for me. I want to be good enough at these areas to know what I know and what I don't, when to bring in the wizards. I'm not sure yet exactly what I'll choose as my area, but it's clear to me that I want to be at the bedside.

By the end of the rotation, I can read ten to twelve echoes a day, and I'm starting to pick up the subtleties. My attendings are complimentary, but not over-the-top. They tell me that I'm mastering the skills, but the reality is that I'm simply less of a novice than I was two weeks ago. I say goodbye to Dr. Millard, and express my gratitude for her teaching. She says it was her pleasure, which takes a long time, but I'm not impatient. I close out the screens on my computer. Tomorrow I leave for Costa Rica—my first break from training in almost a year.

14

COSTA RICA

Reflections on What I'll Be When I Grow Up

Rotations are compartmentalized—end this one; start that one. But they're also cumulative—the impact of one adds to the next. You tell yourself to silo your reactions, but you can't. Sometimes, you need to get away from medicine.

I'm coming off of a combination of bedside and technical rotations. I finish Friday, pack Saturday, drive Sunday, fly from Newark to San José on Monday. By Monday afternoon, I'm on the beach, precisely 2,078 miles from work.

You can begin to think your hospital is the real world, and forget that it's far from it. You get an unrealistic sense of your importance and of where you work. Here no one cares that I'm a doctor, let alone that I work at Hopkins. No matter where you go in the world, medicine—real medicine, local healthcare or lack of it—stares you in the face. Travel to gritty cities and remote locales and you'll find poverty and people for whom some arcane aspect of cardiology is irrelevant. They need clean water and childhood vaccinations to survive. Traveling is a humbling reminder that nuclear stress tests, electrophysiologic ablation, stents, immunosuppressants for transplants, or the fact that I'm a cardiologist are all less important than the need for plain old medicine and good doctors. The Nobel Prize for stem cell therapy can't set a broken arm. More personally, my twelve years of training don't matter if I fail the most basic test of healing. Is that what I want? Is that what I'm choosing?

I'm torn between what I love and what could do the most good. I truly enjoy working with my patients—not just the medical details, but getting to know each person in a way that allows me to understand him or her. And I also enjoy the camaraderie of working as a team, and not only learning from your seniors but, in turn, imparting knowledge to others. And yet, medicine at a distance from one-to-one healing can ultimately effect more change. Research and studies can drive the innovations by which future patients are healed en masse.

Fortunately, medical knowledge has no shortage of applications—in science, business, politics, academics, government. Dr. Sanjay Gupta, trained as a surgeon, now works as an international medical correspondent, exposing and explaining health issues for CNN, a forum so global he reportedly turned down the chance to be U.S. surgeon general. Dr. Bill Frist from Tennessee was a practicing cardiac surgeon who then won a seat in the U.S. Senate. I may not love his politics, but I do like the idea of bringing a medical perspective to public policy. Even my own hiatus from medical training for a degree in public administration was driven by a desire to broaden the application and impact of healthcare knowledge. Men and women trained as doctors employing their medical knowledge in different, unusual, far-reaching ways. That's intriguing to me. Is that what I want?

As clichéd as it sounds, I still don't know what I'll be . . . what my calling is, what subspecialty best suits me. And I seem to be surrounded by people who do know.

I stare at the waves, lie in the sun, and weigh my life choices. . . .

On my plane ride home, I'm trying to enjoy a little nap on board when I hear a thud from the back of the plane. I wish I could just not open my eyes, but I can't help it. Down the aisle, there's a man on the floor, not moving, and a flight attendant hovering over him. I get up and tell the attendant I'm a doctor. The man is a thirty-nine-year-old South American male, an architect, apparently, who'd been heading to the bathroom when he passed out. Now he's awake, confused but semialert. I ask a passenger to vacate a nearby seat and put the man through a cursory neurologic exam, take his vitals, and ask some questions. He has no medical history consistent with the incident—no fainting spells, no chest pain or palpitations, nor is he a diabetic with low blood sugar. He is dehydrated and didn't get much sleep the night before, but these symptoms could be cold- or flu-related. He does not appear to have an infection. The pilot comes back to assess the situation, and I tell him I don't think there's a need to divert the plane but it would be a good idea to have an EMS crew waiting when we land. I go back to my seat, and by then, we're ready to descend. Mentally, I feel as if I'm already back at work. Maybe I never left.

Veteran doctors will tell you that once you choose medicine, you're never away from it. The reality is that it is always there, waiting for you.

15

ROTATION: ECHOCARDIOGRAPHY, PART II

I Get to Drive

Postvacation, it's the first week of March, and I'm headed to Bayview for my second echo rotation.

Echo at Bayview is similar to echo at Hopkins downtown, but there are some key differences. As a smaller hospital with fewer echo studies to interpret, Bayview has only one Fellow per each attending. With the right attending, this can be a great opportunity; with a bad attending, the rotation can be a little painful. I get lucky and draw Dr. Benjamin, an outstanding attending. Dr. Benjamin is in his late thirties, which makes him young for the position. He's in only his third or fourth year as a faculty member, and he did his cardiology fellowship at Hopkins so he knows exactly what I'm going through. He's a work-hard, play-hard guy like me; unlike me, he plays club rugby, and his boxlike shape is built for the rough game. I'm content to stay away from the scrum, but I like his stories. I get a kick out of the visual contradiction: He has the body of a wrestler but the brain of a professor. He's equally at home quoting from Chevy Chase movies or listening to Snoop Dogg while he explores the intricacies of transesophageal echocardiograms. Dr. Benjamin is a total cardiologist, with time in the echo lab, plus time in the CICU as an attending and time as a clinician—but what most interests me about him is that even though he has established himself, in some ways he is still deciding which area he wants to concentrate on or whether he even wants to settle in one area. He's not convinced he'll be a Hopkins "lifer," and regularly mentions how he wants to know what it would be like to practice in a different setting, with different responsibilities and facing different challenges. He brings an unusual perspective to the career choice issue: He's doing what he loves now, but he embraces change in an evolutionary and growth sense, regarding his career as the journey, in motion, rather than set and jelled. It's an intriguing and appealing approach. One more way for me to think about what's next.

For the upcoming two weeks, I will be working alongside Dr. Benjamin on two different kinds of echoes. The TTE, or transthoracic echo, is the standard echo, where gel is put on a patient's chest and then a technician moves the probe around to capture images of the heart. The TEE, or transesophageal echo, is a more invasive echo in which a probe goes into the patient's mouth, down into his or her esophagus, and right behind the heart. These ultrasound images are as close to the heart as you can get without being in it, and although the procedure is more complicated, it can yield more information. The TEE is used when we're worried about an infected heart valve; or a blood clot in one of the chambers; or a "patent foramen ovale," which is a particular kind of connection that exists between the left and right atrium. Essentially, the TEE is a more invasive look for certain kinds of potential problems. Downtown, first-year Fellows don't do them.

But Dr. Benjamin has an almost immediate trust in me, and on my second day, he casually asks if I've performed a TEE before. Even though my response is "Well, not exactly," he keeps going: "You'll be fine. You're good at this stuff." Being asked to assist in doing a TEE without experience is like being thrown in the pool and told you know how to swim; but I can sense that Dr. Benjamin is testing me, and I don't want to pass up the opportunity.

Before we do the TEE, we need to prep the patient with a description of the procedure. My job is to explain what we're going to do, why we're going to do it, how long it will take, and answer any questions the patient might have. The goal is to have an honest discussion about this procedure, but without making it sound like an outtake from a horror film. (I've heard a few prep talks that sounded like a scene from *Friday the 13th*.) I review the risks and benefits, and have the patient or family member sign the informed-consent document for the formal go-ahead.

The patient is Mr. Barlow, a seventy-two-year-old with a litany of heart issues. Today, we're looking to see whether he has any evidence of a blood clot in one of his heart chambers, the left atrium. Although the transesophageal echocardiogram is an invasive procedure, it is made easier by the fact that patients aren't fully awake—they're in conscious sedation, or a "twilight" state. The procedure starts with a series of IV infusions: First, there's Versed, the brand name for midazolam, a sedative in the benzodiazepine class. Then comes fentanyl, an IV opioid narcotic, both a pain and sedating medicine. The two drugs are complementary, making people sleepy enough that they won't be anxious and won't remember much about the procedure itself.

As Mr. Barlow is about to go under, we insert a bite guard with a ring into his mouth. We also spray the back of his mouth with lidocaine, an oral anesthetic, so that the probe will feel less uncomfortable. Inserting the probe is the most difficult part of the TEE: It has to pass into the mouth, through the ring, and down the back of the throat, before it dips down into the esophagus, a tricky path of bends, curves, and nerves and home of the gag reflex. And then I, for the first time in my life, pass the probe. Before inserting the scope, I yell the patient's name to make sure he's asleep: "Mr. Barlow! Mr. Barlow!!" No response, aside from his deep, relaxed breathing. I put the scope in.

I've heard that sometimes, no matter how much lidocaine you put on the back of the throat, no matter how sleepy the patient, the gag reflex is so conditioned, you may never overcome the patient's resistance and get the probe through. And I know if I don't get it on the first or second try, Dr. Benjamin will step in. (Later in the rotation, I see that sometimes even he encounters the gag problem.) But I don't want that to happen on my first TEE. Once I've maneuvered the probe into the patient's throat, there's the central challenge of getting all the views needed, at all the depths and angles. If I don't get them all, again, Dr. Benjamin will have to step in.

I snake the long, thin probe down Mr. Barlow's throat, taking pictures at different angles and depths, guided step-by-step by Dr. Benjamin's calming instructions. At first, it feels strange to operate from the other end of the probe. Dr. Benjamin coaches me through each maneuver, and I move slowly and steadily, following his cues. My hands are on the scope, but there is a sense of security in knowing that he could take over if something goes wrong. Fortunately, nothing does, and Dr. Benjamin never needs to step in.

Once the probe is removed, Mr. Barlow slowly awakens as the sedation wears off, and while we write the report. Even that's different than at Hopkins downtown. There, I viewed the scans on the computer screen and wrote the report in the small, dark room. Here, I performed the procedure myself and saw the results in real time. I'm viewing and mentally writing the report as the test occurs. And perhaps the most impactful difference is that I've been made to feel as if I have real responsibility here. Granted, it's a responsibility overseen by Dr. Benjamin, but I've been given the chance to "do" rather than just "see." I'm accountable. The patient is in my hands. This difference alone makes the rotation considerably more meaningful.

Over the next few days, Dr. Benjamin has me do transesophageal echoes on a regular basis. Working with him makes echo exciting, and it helps me understand echo's important role as the forward line of troops/observation for other doctors. We look for blood clots in the chambers of the heart, because a clot in the left atrium means that a cardioversion (an attempt to get the heart back into normal rhythm) can send the clot traveling up the arterial highway and cause a stroke. We check for infected heart valves, something you can't always see easily on a transthoracic echo—

you need to be as close to the heart as possible to clearly visualize certain valves. When we're not doing transesophageals, we're in the echo lab (listening to Dr. Benjamin's rap music), going through the studies together. This is a rare opportunity to learn. There are thirty to forty transthoracic echoes done at the hospital by the techs each day but only two or three transesophageals, at most. And he trusts me to do them.

I didn't think I'd be saying this after my first echo rotation, but my second echo rotation is truly exciting. From first reading in the morning, to getting TEE consents, to doing them, it is one of the most impactful experiences of my fellowship. And it's all about the contrast: bedside versus textbook, hands-on versus hands-off, patients versus pictures. This rotation is healing. In the largest sense, to me, this is medicine.

One TEE is particularly memorable, to put it mildly. Garrett is a young utility lineman, burned during what was supposed to be a routine job. He now lies in the burn intensive care unit, with third-degree burns on more than 50 percent of his face, chest, and arms. I've never seen anything like it, frankly, almost monstrous. He's attached to a breathing machine, and because of the damage to his skin (normally a protective barrier between our bodies and the outside world, keeping infections and toxins out), he's now fighting major issues with infection. The ICU doctors need us to determine whether Garrett has an infected heart valve. They also need any evidence we can find of heart failure, because on top of everything else, related or not to his burns, he is now experiencing low blood pressure.

First, we have to get permission from Garrett's family.

This is one of those medical situations where each procedure is only one small piece in the patient's total, complex, multi-layered condition and care. Even so, the family's first question is, "Is this test going to get him better?" This is a difficult question to answer. Tests don't make people better. If he gets better, it will be over time, with myriad treatments for the myriad interrelated consequences of his body's burns. The real answer to the family's question is that doing the TEE won't make him better, but failing to look for an infected heart valve could kill him. Instead, I reply, "Checking his heart valve is a necessary step in treating Garrett's overall condition so that he can begin the healing process. . . ." The family gives us the go.

The indelible imprint from this experience is the human one. We doctors are sometimes expected to act as emotionless scientists. Examine, probe, go in, do your procedure, get the information, operate, implant, remove, medicate, write in the chart, send the patient home, see the next one. . . . But sometimes, on a purely human level, a patient's condition is just so sad, awful, and unfair—and we feel it as much as anyone. This poor man looks like a horrific casualty of war, and his physical pain is palpable. It hurts to see his family see his pain. And now we have to shove a probe down his throat. As I pass the probe, I try to get a sense as to whether I'm causing Garrett any additional discomfort, but it's impossible to know. Everything about his current appearance screams discomfort. He's sedated, on a breathing machine, with burns that make him appear as fragile as any patient I've ever met. Move by move, we get the pictures we need, as gently as possible, trying not to disturb him. Thankfully, the test shows that there's no valve infection. But the Hippocratic oath's implicit dictum does run through my mind as I do the test. "Do no harm." Are we following it or violating it? It's a wrenching case for me and even for veterans such as Dr. Benjamin.

Some aspects of medicine are exercises of skill; some, of mind; a few, of both. The real crux of medical acumen is often the combination of the test results and the action—what you know and what you do with it. The attending can point to where you need work, to what will make you more adept at performing a test or at reading it, or to a technique or tip, or even back to an early classroom lesson. Your job is to go where he or she points and do it.

16

ROTATION: CARDIAC CATHETERIZATION— INTERVENTIONAL CARDIOLOGY

The Closest We Get to Being Surgeons

Mind shift: another first day of another rotation, this time from the predictability of echo to the pressures of the cath lab. This is an eight-week rotation, all of it intense. The patients cover a wide spectrum, from those in for outpatient procedures because something is suspected to be wrong, to the emergencies in need of a cath immediately because something is known to be very wrong right now. As a resident, I'd been around cath and observed (from the other side of the glass), but now I will have the chance not just to watch but to do it. It's highly specialized, the territory of the interventional cardiologists, who do one thing—invasive cardiac procedures. It's as close to heart surgery as you can get without sawing open the sternum. You're going directly into blood vessels, inserting devices that open jammed arteries to let blood flow through to dying heart muscle, immediately saving a life or prolonging it.

Cath is the sexier, higher-octane side of cardiology. But after a while, even the most miraculous-seeming procedures can be broken down to the basics—as mechanical, electrical, or chemical repairs. They're each logical and practical, even if uncommon . . . including cath. I'll deconstruct the procedure to see how it works and then go about conquering a new skill.

In contrast to some previous rotations, in cath I won't be learning the procedure exclusively from one individual attending with whom I might bond or whom I might know from previous experience. There are ten different interventional attendings, and on any given day, two or three are doing caths. They are each impressive, but each quite different in teaching style and demeanor. The way you learn or how much you learn is highly dependent upon which attending is in the lab that day. A case in point is Dr. Calvin, in his midforties, a relative newcomer given the decade plus of medical training it takes to get where he is. He's patient and soft-spoken, which is also notable because it belies the stereotype for such hotshots. Dr. Calvin seems to have trained his reactions to be the inverse of the situation, low-stress in high-stress circumstances. He's excellent to work with because you feel you can do no wrong, or rather that he'll enable you to feel you can do no wrong, and in case you do, he'll calmly fix it.

Dr. Calvin starts with the elementary aspects, how to hold and manipulate the catheters. As a first-timer, my role as the Fellow is to "get access," or insert the initial catheter into the femoral artery. Then, during the remainder of the procedure, I assist. Getting access can be unpredictable. You may get it right away . . . or not. Some of the attendings give you one or two tries, then step in and say, "Let me take it now," and you feel lousy, especially when they stick the catheter in as if the artery were as wide as the Amazon.

On day three, my first turn comes. I make my attempt, but I don't get it. Dr. Calvin just nods at me to make my next try. I miss again. He offers a pointer on how to guide the catheter. I get it. He says, "Not that hard, is it?" Instead of feeling lousy, I feel good. Pretty basic psychology, but pretty effective. The next two cases, I get in on the first try.

My experience is very different from the story circulating about another Fellow who took two tries, whose attending actually bodychecked him aside and didn't give him another opportunity for weeks, by which time the Fellow was convinced he had artery blindness.

I hit plenty of arteries and miss a few, but I start to feel I'm catching on. Two weeks in, I'm working with another attending, this one not known for his tolerance. I have a patient whose femoral artery pulse I can't find, which means I can't tell where to stick the catheter needle. In this case, the man has a lot of "soft tissue" in the groin area where we go in; he's substantially overweight. After I miss on the first try, today's attending is literally breathing down my neck. I do not panic. Instead, I channel Dr. Calvin—patience and calm—feel around the excess flesh to be extrasensitive to the pulse, take my time, find the pulse . . . and go right into the artery. The heavy breathing behind me subsides.

I have my off days, of course. Around the third week, I'm zero for four on one patient. Dr. Calvin lets me keep going for a fifth and even a sixth try. Finally, in sympathy for the patient, and without destroying my ego, he says, "This one is tough. Mind if I give it a shot?" The next day I get the first one on the first try. It takes practice.

But the veterans seem to be able to get access every time. One of the older interventionists, Dr. Zachary, is beyond good—almost legendary. A former Vietnam Green Beret, cool under fire, Dr. Zachary is known to offer a dry joke when the situation is tense. My first time with him, I'm not hitting the artery. Almost inaudibly, he says, "Take your time, Dan. We have nothing else to do today." It's his style, but it can throw you. Later that day, while trying to find the pulse, I say, "I can feel it." He replies, "That's great. But the point is to be inside the artery. Let us know when you're in there." Battlefield humor, but with a point—get on with the procedure; there's a patient who needs it and another doctor waiting for the results.

Around week three, I get a message on my pager that has nothing to do with cath. A second-year resident, one of the best in her class, and applying for a cardiology fellowship, is about to submit her rank list to the National Resident Matching Program. She wants to hear how I made my final decision. And, it turns out, we have a shared experience.

After a bit of self-conscious hemming and hawing, she reveals that she has come down to a mental tie between Hopkins and Harvard/Brigham and that she's been contacted by each telling her she's at the top of both of their match lists. When I share with her that I had a similar experience, she breathes an audible sigh of relief. She was reluctant to tell me for fear of sounding immodest. I confide in her that while, on the one hand, it was a wonderful choice to have to make, at the same time, it left me almost unable to decide. She has managed to stumble upon someone who can empathize.

I try my best not to tell her what to do but to frame the issue so she can decide wisely. On the pure cardiology side of the equation, either institution is superb, renowned, staffed with incredible doctors, equipped with state-of-the-art facilities and research. So I suggest she look at the nonmedical side. She's a graduate of Stanford medical school, a second-generation Hispanic American, from a high-achieving family. Where does her family live? Is there someone significant in her life? Where might she want to live after training? Her family is in a suburb of Philadelphia, not far from Hopkins, and they're close. She's in a relationship with another doctor who is finishing a family medicine residency in Cleveland, about to go somewhere as yet undetermined. Hopkins is a powerful force. But she's been at Hopkins; it's like home, for better or worse. And Harvard is . . . Harvard, the biggest "brand" in academia. One other thing Harvard has is Boston, a great city. At Hopkins, we always have to say, "Baltimore is nicer than you think." What Hopkins has is the medicine, second to none. She doesn't have to decide today, but soon, within two weeks. The only advice I offer is to do not what lines up on paper but what "feels right."

(*Update:* Three weeks later, I get a message from her: "I'm coming to Hopkins. Thanks for listening.")

I'm at the halfway point of cath, and two lessons emerge. The first is "the contradiction." Interventionalists (and occasionally other specialists) are sometimes nicknamed "procedure monkeys" by their peers because they're highly trained to perform a single feat, almost to the exclusion of all else, and therefore could seem to possess very little humanity. Therein lies the contradiction. Often the attending who can be all-business—callous, or sarcastic, or temperamental, or unforgiving toward Fellows who miss arteries—is the same attending who displays the most sensitive, poignant bedside manner with patients and families. These doctors are human when they most need to be. It shatters an accepted prejudice. If you have ice water in your veins when you're under fire, you must be ice-cold all the time. Not so. What isn't clear is how these doctors got that way.

In all of medical training, there's no course or rotation called "bedside manner" ... despite the fact that we may spend half of our days at bedsides. No one teaches you how to deliver a diagnosis, or treatment plan, or surgical outcome, or prognosis, or news of death to patients and families. You learn by watching. Or not. And after the case is over, there's no review of those skills, no reflection, no "What did we learn, and how can we do it better?" The assumption is, we'll learn it out of necessity. Good bedside manner isn't just good care, it's good business. It should be taught.

The second lesson is not as surprising: You learn differently from different attendings, depending on their styles, patience levels, and amount of leeway they give the Fellow. Personally, I like Dr. Zachary, despite his hardened exterior, but some Fellows don't. My gauge of an attending is whether he or she (a) pushes me, (b) shows me something new, (c) isn't dull. Dr. Zachary does all three. Another attending, Dr. Delano, is crotchety, anal, and controlling, but if you can tolerate his manner, he can impart some valuable cath lessons.

The bottom line is, they don't all "teach" in the textbook sense; some just do what they do, the way they've always done it, and it's up to the Fellows to figure out how to extract the lessons . . . even if it practically requires surgery.

And then there are actually some attendings you'd rather not learn from.

Given a choice . . .

By weeks five and six, I am getting better at caths. Early in the fellowship, people asked me if I was going into cath as a career. Everyone has heard of caths; famous people get them; they're in the news. The truth is, doing caths sounds exciting, like flying in the space shuttle, but in reality, who knows?

Until a month ago, I had seen caths but never done one. When you're a resident, you can go to the cath lab and sit in the control room behind the thick glass and view the procedure on screens. But you might as well be watching the Discovery Channel. It's a lot different from being in the room and passing the catheter into an artery, or missing and sweating beneath your mask.

Now I'm doing them, going from virgin to immersion in a matter of days. With some attendings, it's a good immersion, and with others, not so good, and you don't have much choice. But there is one guy I'd like to avoid: Dr. Rutherford. I had a negative experience with him as a resident, coincidentally in a cath-related clinical situation.

I was the resident on call in the cardiac ICU, on a thirty-hour shift. Mr. Robbins, a patient with unstable angina, had come in, was cathed in the evening, stented in two major coronary arteries, and admitted to the cardiac ICU. At 2:00 a.m., I was summoned to his bedside because he was having an active groin bleed. He'd called the nurse because he felt something warm on his leg—and it turned out to be blood. From the site where they had gone in with the catheter, a half liter of bright red was squirting onto his bedsheets. The situation wasn't complicated: Unless immediate pressure is applied, the patient can bleed out and die. It's not sophisticated treatment; but it's physically demanding, and it works. The cath Fellow wasn't around, so I had to do it myself. I applied pressure to Mr. Robbins for a solid twenty minutes. The bleeding stopped. Afterward, I paged the Fellow, but he didn't call back, probably because he was sleeping.

The patient was fine, good pulses in his feet, and we had no concern for other vascular damage. We had Mr. Robbins lie flat for the rest of the night to ensure he healed up appropriately and checked his blood counts regularly to make sure he didn't need a transfusion to replace the lost blood.

The next morning I was on rounds with the CICU team—the ICU attending, the residents, and the interns. That's when Dr. Rutherford, the interventional attending, appeared. As is the protocol, we stopped everything to discuss this case. Without a hello, he fired at me, "What happened with Mr. Robbins last night?" I recounted the events. "He had a bleed from his puncture site, about four hundred cubic centimeters of blood, discovered by the patient and his nurse. I held twenty minutes of pressure, and there was no subsequent bleeding or hematoma after that." A by-the-book answer. Rather than ask anything further about the treatment, Dr. Rutherford homed in on a technicality: "Why is there no event note in the chart?" An event note is a documented record that recounts an unexpected incident with a patient. Event notes exist, to a great extent, for legal purposes. But Dr. Rutherford was relentless and condescending: "You've got to write an event note in that situation." I hadn't slept for a day and a half, needed a shower, and most important, I was confident I'd done the right thing for the patient, so I was in no frame of mind to be lectured on event notes. But Dr. Rutherford repeated it once more. Rather than being thanked, I felt scolded.

My CICU attending was a very good doctor, but evidently averse to confrontation, so it was up to me to look out for myself. I responded, "Now that the patient is fine, it would be my pleasure to write an event note. I did page your Fellow at 2:30 a.m., so you may want to let him know everything is okay, because he still hasn't called me back and it's now 10:30 a.m." Dr. Rutherford grunted and walked away. That afternoon, before going home to bed, I wrote a two-and-a-half-page event note, recounting in meticulous detail what had occurred.

Dr. Rutherford strikes me as the type who can be fine when all is calm, but when there's stress, he can obsess over details instead of focusing on the key issue, not a good trait for anyone who deals with pressure—a fireman, a cop, an astronaut, or a doctor. Honestly, given a choice, I'd rather not cath with him.

So far I haven't cathed with him, and I won't today because it's 5:30 p.m. Time to clean up, change my shirt, and make sure there are no coffee stains on my tie. This is a big night.

*   *   *

Tonight is Johns Hopkins Medical School graduation. Not only are degrees conferred, but awards are given to students and faculty, one of which is voted on by the graduating class. Across all specialties—surgery, medicine, pediatrics—the students select the resident who has contributed the most to their education. In February, during my consult month, I'd been notified it was me. I'm very flattered.

In contrast to my own graduation, instead of sitting with the 130 people about to walk across the stage, I'm one of the people on the stage, one row back from the CEO of Hopkins Medicine and right behind the commencement speaker, Dr. Denton Cooley, one of the deities of cardiac surgery. My parents insisted on coming for my ten seconds in the spotlight—unfortunately for them, sandwiched into the middle of the three-hour ceremony.

It was worth the entire evening to hear Dr. Cooley. "It feels like just yesterday that I was in your seats, graduating a mere sixty-five years ago." The crowd laughed but got the message. He might be almost ninety, but he's as sharp as ever. His speech was fatherly and wise. Work earnestly and ignore the naysayers. He exhorts young doctors to do what they're passionate about, not just what's lucrative or the newest flavor. What makes the speech powerful is his passion, the passion he's maintained for over half a century. He leaves the graduates feeling that if they choose an easy path, he'll be personally disappointed. And you don't want to disappoint this legend who performed the first successful human heart transplant in the United States, and the first implantation of an artificial heart in the world, whose teams have performed more than one hundred thousand cardiac procedures (hence, the title of his memoir: *100,000 Hearts*), who has won every imaginable award, including the Presidential Medal of Freedom; and, not coincidentally, he graduated from the Johns Hopkins School of Medicine.

An hour into the evening, it was time for my award. The CEO of Hopkins Medicine made the announcement and shook my hand; the vice president handed me a framed certificate; and my parents were proud.

But the effect of Dr. Cooley's speech, on the night I received the award, was profound. This medical icon put it in perspective. You got a nice honor tonight. Keep at it and someday you might truly accomplish something. This award says that I do what I do pretty well. Dr. Cooley said, in effect, that it's just a start.

Back to cath for the home stretch—the final two weeks. Put simply, more caths, more practice, more hits, a few misses, more learning, more subtleties. As it turns out, I never had to cath with Dr. Rutherford. Maybe he didn't want to cath with me either.

Cath is over. All in all, I like it. Again, I have to say, I don't know if this is the one thing I want to do every day, forever. It scares me sometimes to think maybe that one thing doesn't exist. Maybe it won't have to be "one thing." Maybe things I like, such as cath, can be in the mix. I don't have to check that box yet. But I will. . . .

17

WEEKEND COVERAGE

A Virtual Two-Day Rotation

On weekends, you push the rotation "pause" button from Friday until Monday. Then, you either have two days off or you have "coverage," meaning duty at one of the hospitals in the system, in one particular department.

In the middle of the cath rotation, I cover the Bayview CICU one weekend, and the experience turns out to be the equivalent of an entire rotation in forty-eight hours. Sometimes you can take in as much in two days as you do in two months.

Friday afternoon, I go to the Bayview CICU and get a sign-out—the list of seven patients and their conditions—from the Fellow heading out for the weekend. My job is to make sure those seven, plus whoever comes in the door, get through the next two days. Monday morning, I'll pass the baton to whichever Fellow is on.

The better part of that Saturday is routine, rounding with the residents in the morning, putting plans in place for the patients in the afternoon, and fielding new patients as they come in. Technically, I can leave at any time the pace allows, as long as I'm prepared to come back. This weekend, I end up never leaving.

For the first several hours, I stay just to get to know a new group of patients, and because the resident on that evening is the competent-but-nervous type, which concerns me. At about 9:30 p.m., I decide I can leave in another fifteen minutes. At 9:45 p.m., the resident gets a call about a patient that the ER wants to send up to the cardiac ICU. She gets off the phone and says, "It might be helpful if you came with me," which means: "Don't leave." On the way downstairs, she tells me about the patient: a sixty-six-year-old woman in the ER critical care bay who has a heart rate of thirty . . . barely life-sustaining. They had applied a temporary transcutaneous pacemaker to her chest to try to pace her heart faster, to get her blood pressure up. (When your heart rate is low, unless you've been training for cross-country, your blood pressure will also be low.) There are several reasons a sixty-six-year-old's heart rate could be thirty, but they are all bad.

Downstairs in the ER, lying in a bed, we see Bunny, a classic, hard-living, beer-drinking, beehived "Hon"—what the locals call certain other locals, born and bred in Baltimore, often with big hair and a heavy accent. Next to her is her identical twin sister—same hair, same accent. Bunny is pale as a ghost, awake but confused, disoriented, and irritated—and, she says, exhausted.

Behind a curtain in the bay, I coax a coherent story out of her with some help from her sister. In the past two days, she's gone from feeling like her old self to feeling as if she were carrying the weight of the world, and nothing relieves it. On her Saturday errands, she can normally walk the two blocks to the grocery store, carrying her bags or pushing them in a cart. But today she couldn't even get herself down the stairs to the door. Realizing something is wrong, she calls an ambulance, and when they arrive, with her heart rate of thirty, conscious but woozy, she offers the patient go-to description, "I feel crappy."

Now we have to find out what's going on and why. Is it a heart attack? Is it from medicine she's taking, perhaps in excess? Is it more mysterious? In a purely academic sense, this is a beautiful medical case (as in the art of solving a medical mystery). There are four challenges ahead of us. First, get Bunny out of the emergency room. Nothing good happens in the ER after thirty minutes. ER doctors are conditioned to be at their best right now—fight the fire, defuse the bomb, jerk the shoulder back into the socket, pound the chest, pull the tongue out of the throat, in the moment, but that moment rarely lasts more than thirty minutes. After that, unless the patient is threatening to die, the ER docs move to the next disaster. The second challenge is to make sure Bunny is stabilized. She has various devices attached: EKG leads on her chest, as well as pacing pads, one on the front, one on her back, all of which are keeping her heart rate steady. She isn't getting big shocks from a defibrillator but rather mini-jolts every second to get her heart rate to sixty instead of thirty. She's paced; that is, she has blood pressure . . . for now. The third challenge is to make sure Bunny has the attention of doctors, in a monitored setting, because she is clearly sick for reasons we don't yet understand.

That leaves the big challenge, figuring out the "why." I have never faced this exact type of case before, but I have now had an almost yearlong crash course in seeing people who have something wrong with their hearts and unraveling the mystery. You develop a detective's instinct and methodology— a deductive process to go through the algorithms and arrive at initial conclusions, remain calm, and avoid panic. That's the difference between July of last year and April of this year—the difference between a resident and a Fellow.

We transport Bunny upstairs to the cardiac ICU and continue to deal with the challenge of stabilization. Being paced through the chest is not a good long-term plan—usually, a transcutaneous pacemaker is used only for short periods of time as a bridge to another step—because the device can stop working and because it's uncomfortable for the patient. The more definitive way is to place a transvenous pacing wire, which is done by inserting a large IV into the patient's neck and floating a temporary pacing wire down the vein in her neck into the right atrium of her heart, crossing the tricuspid valve into the right ventricle, where the wire sits in the muscle and can pace the heart directly. It sounds invasive, but once the wire is in place, it's considerably more comfortable for the patient, because the amount of electricity required to pace the heart from within the heart is far lower than the amount needed to travel from an exterior pad through the chest.

This procedure—inserting the transvenous pacing wire—is not done frequently. And I've never done it. I have to make the decision—there's no attending present to make the call for me—and I have to decide fast. I weigh the data. In the ER, they drew blood and sent it for analysis. Now, forty-five minutes later, the test results come in and might suggest an explanation. Bunny's blood counts are normal, including the white blood count, meaning it's probably not a raging infection. However, her electrolyte panel shows substantial indications of acute renal failure. Her kidneys, though not functioning at zero, are much worse than when she last visited the clinic. The red flag is the level of potassium (K) in her blood. The heart relies on normal levels of potassium—not too much or too little—to conduct and function properly. Normal K level is between 3.5 and 5.0 (lab measurement units). The 5.0 to 6.0 range will get the attention of the clinic doctor; above 6.0, you need to be in the hospital. Over 6.5 and you're flirting with danger. Bunny's is 7.2—trouble. There'd been a delay from the lab on her K number because it had to be double-checked, and whenever there's a double check, you can bet the number isn't going to be normal. Okay, her 7.2 makes some sense; her slow rhythms are almost certainly from potassium overload. Probable conclusion: Fix the K; don't put in the wire.

Before I rule out the wire option, though, I want to talk to the attending. My instinct says that Bunny is being paced through the skin and she's not terribly uncomfortable. On the other hand, putting in a pacing wire is a central line procedure, meaning floating a wire down into somebody's heart, and that can lead to complications, puncturing the wall, maybe causing an arrhythmia. But I need to vet my conclusion, because my N (numerical sample size of experience) is currently zero. I call my attending at home and say, "Sorry to wake you, but here's the situation. . . ." I walk him through the case and my conclusion, and he says, "I concur completely." More important, he doesn't say, "Two hours from now, check in and let me know what happens." He trusts my take. (I could have made the decision without his blessing, but I wanted to run it by him that night to vet it, and I want to teach the resident the right way to do things.)

It's now 12:45 a.m. We have to get the potassium level down. There are only a couple of basic ways for the body to physiologically get rid of things: urinate or defecate. There's also vomit, but it's not preferred by patient or doctor. One route, despite Bunny's sick kidneys, is a large dose—eighty milligrams—of the IV diuretic Lasix. The other route is a nasty-tasting medicine called Kayexalate, which gets the bowels to eliminate potassium from the GI tract. Given the severity of Bunny's condition, she gets both. The Kayexalate takes a while, but with the IV Lasix, we hope to see a response fast. And even with her renal function at 15 percent of normal, within forty-five minutes, she is urinating into a Foley catheter, about five hundred cubic centimeters, or half a liter. We send off another blood test for potassium.

We're reasonably confident of the results because we'd done a short-term maneuver to, at least temporarily, move the potassium from the blood cells into tissues. We'd used an IV cocktail of calcium and insulin, plus sugar, or dextrose (so the insulin doesn't make the sugar drop and cause hypoglycemia). With that combo, Bunny's heart rate had come up right away and didn't require as much pacing . . . but that effect will last only until the cocktail is out of her system and the body reverts to its previous state. The temporary result was a clue that we're on the right track.

I use the blood test waiting time to think a few steps ahead, a now-ingrained behavior from fellowship. If this works, okay, but if not, then what? The most surefire way to de-K patients is to dialyze them. At midnight, I tell the resident, "Call renal to discuss the case because we may have to do an emergency dialysis session." I could call the kidney doctors myself, but the resident needs both the experience and the middle-of-the-night pushback; it's all part of her training.

Within the hour, the renal team arrives and puts a dialysis catheter in Bunny's femoral vein. Her potassium level comes from the lab, and it's 6.5—down but still high. As quickly as we take the potassium out of her system, it seems to come back (which is a clue to what triggered it in the first place but we don't know that yet). There's still not enough progress. I speak to the kidney doctors about readying the dialysis machine.

In the meantime, we give Bunny an additional 120 milligrams of Lasix. This time she puts out about eight hundred cubic centimeters of urine, almost a full liter. We test again sixty minutes later, and her potassium is down to 5.9. The dialysis isn't needed yet. If a sick kidney is making urine, it's probably getting better. An hour later, Bunny's K level is down to 5.5. Her EKG shows she's generating her own rhythm—heart rate at sixty-five—no longer totally reliant on the pacer. We turn the pacer off, and Bunny's heart rate remains at sixty-five. Her blood pressure is coming up too. It's 3:30 in the morning.

Bunny's body is sending out cautiously optimistic signals. She was ash white; now she has a little color. She wasn't able to communicate well; now she speaks in full sentences. Her sister and her girlfriends see the difference. Medically, her potassium is coming down, and she's generating a heart rhythm on her own. What the textbooks say should happen is happening.

One last potassium check: 5.3, trend line in the right direction. At 4:00 a.m., I leave, seven hours later than I expected. Driving home, I wonder: If I hadn't stayed that extra fifteen minutes, and if the same events had transpired, would the resident have called me?

And one other question haunts me: "How did Bunny's potassium get so high?" That question is there, still unsolved, but it will wait, and can wait, until morning.

Unfortunately, morning comes just a few hours later, at 7:00 a.m. Bunny is still in her own rhythm. Her potassium is in the 4s, normal for anybody. She's essentially weaned off the blood pressure–supporting medicine. All good. Since her K is now down, the resident asks, "Did we put the dialysis catheter in unnecessarily?" I reply, "Absolutely not. We did the safe thing by being prepared to dialyze her the moment her potassium inched up rather than having to spend an hour and a half getting it in later, when she might have been truly vulnerable."

Now we need to answer the "How did the K get so high in the first place?" question. If Bunny had suffered through her symptoms one more night at home, she likely would have arrested and died, with the death perhaps chalked up to "natural causes"—which, given what we subsequently find out, would not have been natural at all.

We search through Bunny's medical records, reconstructing events. She has a baseline history of some congestive heart failure and a propensity to retain fluid. To combat it, she was on a diuretic, oral Lasix, to keep fluids balanced and the heart appropriately unloaded. She'd seen her primary care doctor three weeks before, and her blood work showed that her kidneys were functioning at only 70 percent, which was new for her. Her doctor concluded she was getting too much diuretic, which can dehydrate, and with dehydration, the kidneys can start to shut down. The doctor then, logically, decided to substantially cut back the dose of the diuretic. But what *wasn't* addressed was the fact that, like many people on diuretics, Bunny was also on oral potassium to compensate for the potassium she was urinating. Her doctor cut the oral diuretic but didn't cut the potassium. So when Bunny continued to take her supplemental potassium, together with other medications that raise potassium levels, she accumulated it in her system until it caused a disaster. Unfortunately, this information was not in her records since her primary care doctor is not in the Hopkins system.

But Bunny actually helped us piece it together, in a way. She proved one of the two rules attributed to an apocryphal resident, way back when. Rule 1: Patients always lie, whether they mean to or not. Rule 2: When patients are too sick to lie, their families will lie for them, again purposefully or not. What the rules mean is that usually without any intention to mislead, people tend to present the facts selectively or even falsely, either because they want to look like good, conscientious patients, or because they don't want to present bad news, or because their memories are limited, or some combination of all those elements. As a result, the lore goes, you can't rely on what patients and their families say. You have to listen past the words, to what was not said.

This woman told us she had taken a diuretic, but she didn't tell us the dosage had been reduced, nor did her sister. And she didn't mention the potassium at all. But in our search for whatever we didn't know, what might not have been told to us, her sister did give us the name of Bunny's primary care doctor and had his office send us her records. There was a note saying, "Diuretic likely causing dehydration and lower kidney function. Cut back diuretic." Attached was also a list of medications, including the potassium, but no notation to lower the potassium dosage. And we found that she was also on a blood pressure medicine that can, in the event of kidney failure, make the patient more likely to have high potassium.

Mystery solved. Good outcome for the patient; good learning for me and for the resident. Even in situations where I don't immediately have the answers, I'm developing a set of skills that enable me to cope with whatever presents itself. I have a sense of being outside myself, watching myself handle a challenge. And I'm pleased. That may sound cocky, but it's not. It's a relief. It's good to know that the clinical training we're getting is working.

Early Monday morning, I do the return handoff to the CICU Fellow, after my two-day cram rotation in the Bayview CICU, and go back to finish up cath.

18

ROTATION: PREVENTIVE CARDIOLOGY, PART II

Working with the Guru

I'm ready to start preventive . . . but it turns out preventive begins with me. After a two-day break for mountain climbing in a New Hampshire hailstorm, I report to my rotation hacking and dripping. A nurse spots my symptoms and sends me to the ER for a flu swab, which means sitting and waiting like any other patient, which is a good empathy experience, but I wouldn't mind being taken to the front of the line. Finally, I'm released with a diagnosis of a "cold," and instructions to try not to sneeze on anyone.

With almost a year of fellowship behind me, I'm a different doctor on my second preventive rotation than on the first, but one thing is the same: the attending, Dr. Franklin, the preventive guru.

I meet him at Hopkins downtown at 8:00 a.m. in the outpatient center. We hit the day full throttle with a packed panel of patients. I see five; he sees my five plus another six of his own. The morning is vintage Dr. Franklin. In three and a half hours, he talks to every patient, adjusts his or her cholesterol medicine, checks the patient's progress, and does whatever he can to prevent a heart attack, all the while marketing himself and his field.

In preventive cardiology at Hopkins, he is the brand. The world knows it and comes to consult him. This morning we see a sitting member of Congress, unnamed but of *Meet the Press* level; then the chairman of the board of trustees at an Ivy League school; then the former chair of a medical department at Hopkins, now head of an international healthcare consulting firm (Franklin is a doctor's doctor); then the founder/CEO of a defense-contracting conglomerate in northern Virginia. The CEO is sixty, responsible for a billion-dollar enterprise; his board and shareholders are betting a lot on his body and heart, so there's only one guy to see. The list goes on. Some people are famous, some are rich, some both, but what they have in common is Dr. Franklin, the master. He doesn't ask just about their heart; he asks about their business, or the government, or their golf game. It's a studied but effective form of personal interaction. And the celebrity aspect can't help but be enticing.

Personally, I find it a little uncomfortable dealing with patients who think they're important. But Dr. Franklin seems to be able to shoot the breeze and yet maintain attention, focus, and objectivity. Not everyone can do that. These people are used to being treated differently, and that can be dangerous, even affecting the quality of service. We're all human. If Bruce Springsteen walks in, we're going to say, "Holy shit, it's the Boss," and want to text everyone we know. Even Dr.

Franklin is a bit of a stargazer, but he also seems like a star himself. His office is a photo gallery of Dr. Franklin and Somebody Famous.

Monday of week two, our first patient is a venture capitalist who splits his time between Silicon Valley and Maryland's Eastern Shore, travels two hundred days a year, meeting clients and making deals, but doesn't take time to stay in shape and now gets winded going up a flight of stairs. His primary care doctor discovered he has high blood pressure and high cholesterol and tells him to see a cardiologist. Who else but Dr. Franklin?

At lunchtime, I walk outside and am reminded of the Big Contrast. In East Baltimore, people are living marginal lives, some with drug problems, some working hard but barely making it, most with little or no health insurance. And all the while, shahs, politicos, and honchos are being escorted through Hopkins's doors. The contrast is stark. And unfair.

I ask myself, if I attain some level of success professionally and financially, will I maintain the compassion to care for the person whose life is unlike mine? I can do it at thirty, but could I still at fifty? I see colleagues—with good values— who seem to grow callous, or at least resigned to realities they can't change. The system has made it harder to take care of the disadvantaged, uninformed, uninsured person. It may be spiritually fulfilling, but there's little upside, and plenty of downside—financial, time, prestige—for the hospital, for doctors, for the healthcare system. Is the poor person less deserving of good care than the affluent? Of course not, but it's a challenge. And it's amazing—and revealing—how grateful people are when they're treated with dignity, having gone through much of life without it. It's equally amazing, and upsetting, how often the overprivileged may take good care for granted. I try to be as understanding of the tanned, rich scion as of the average Joe. Both have the same physiology inside, the same heart disease. Both need the same tests, the same drugs, the same stents or surgery. One of the takeaways from preventive is to ask the identical questions, try to react the identical way, stay focused on the medical issues, not celebrity, golf games, or airplanes. There's a credibility you gain by not treating patients as if they're special, but by going right to matters of health. Treat them all as patients—the average guy, the poor, the rich, the star—all just people, sick or worried about getting sick. They are people who are scared and want care.

I confess to a prejudice right now in favor of the disadvantaged, or at least in favor of pushing for a level playing field in how we treat patients. Maybe that will erode over time and I will become callous. I hope not.

It's 11:45 a.m., Wednesday, June 10, and I'm driving to White Marsh clinic, mentally replaying an incident yesterday at the diabetes clinic. Senior endocrinologists run the clinic, but the role of cardiologists there is to get people better from a diabetic standpoint, which, in turn, can help get them better from a cardiovascular standpoint. Diabetes, along with high blood pressure, smoking, and a few other villains, is at the top of the list of risk factors for development of coronary artery disease. Treating a root cause can, to some extent, treat the entire equation.

But the case I see is emblematic of why, in many patient populations, preventing cardiovascular disease before it happens is an uphill battle. The patient, Ms. Bailey, is sixty-two, not old by today's medical standards, African American, lives in East Baltimore, has children who bring her groceries, but is otherwise on her own (a sharp contrast to the VIPs). When I walk into her room, she's in a wheelchair, best guess about five foot six, 250 pounds, talking with her forehead in her hand, eyes closed. After missing several appointments with her primary care doctor, she had mounting calamities by the time she saw him—high cholesterol, high blood pressure, plus diabetes, and sleep apnea due to obesity—and he sent her to the clinic.

My one mission is to talk about Ms. Bailey's diabetes, not her other problems, and it takes discipline to keep her on point. No matter the question, she talks about her chronic pain—which is understandable, but not what we're here for. I ask how often she takes her insulin. "Twice a day. In the morning and after lunch." Not good. It should be in the morning and evening. I ask, "What time after lunch?" She says, "Actually, it's before dinner." I ask, "Is it closer to after lunch or before dinner?" She holds her head and says, "I don't know, maybe before dinner." I finally learn she takes her insulin at 9:00 in the morning and around 6:00 in the evening, give or take. That would be okay because it's a twelve-hour formulation, but I get the strong sense she is hardly consistent. She's on a long list of other medicines, but similarly, we don't know if she's taking those regularly or not. I ask her directly, "How often do you forget to take your insulin?" She says, "Oh, a lot . . . a real lot." I say, "Ms. Bailey, this morning did you take your insulin?" Her answer is "I don't remember." She has no diagnosis of dementia; she's conversing; she got herself to the clinic. She's just not capable, from a cognitive standpoint, of taking care of her own illnesses.

I have to wonder what we can do to lower Ms. Bailey's risk of long-term damage from the disease when she's having so much trouble in the short term. She is a statistical case study, one patient with multiple risk factors that add up to comorbidities, or potential ways to die. The system hasn't totally failed Ms. Bailey. In fact, it is trying to reach out to her, but in doing so, it has overwhelmed her with a long list of medications and directions that she can't keep straight. She lives alone, on government disability, likely to be increasingly debilitated, with almost no social support in the way of family or friends to help with her meds, her weight, and life's other challenges.

It hits me hard: Despite all of the high-tech tools at our disposal, it takes a willing and capable patient, plus outside support. Without those components, nothing works. Preventive cardiology? Preventive anything? How about just staying alive? There are countless people in urban America, like the locals in Colombia or Costa Rica or anywhere else, who need a basic doctor and basic support more than they need any specialist, cardiovascular or otherwise.

That's what I'm thinking as I pull into the parking lot of the upwardly mobile, suburban White Marsh clinic. The average patients here aren't average at all. They're aware and have families and access to Googled information and insurance, and they're generally motivated to get better. Another study in contrasts.

The last day of the preventive rotation, Dr. Franklin gives

a lunchtime talk to the Fellows. He says his goal is nothing less than to change human behavior so that heart disease happens less. A challenging and noble goal. Realistic? Highest priority? I'm not so sure. Not nearly as sure as I might have been twelve months ago.

19

365 DAYS A FELLOW

What I Learned

After preventive, I have one more rotation, part III of echocardiography, a return to the sequestered caves of echo, essentially a repeat of parts I and II—venerated but narrow practitioners, nuanced/vague interpretations of pictures, via imperfect technology—a reminder of a highly specialized field I do not wish to pursue.

Echo is followed by a weekend in the cardiac ICU, featuring a refresher course in "the groin hold." An eighty-two-year-old frail but fleshy woman has had a cardiac catheterization via her femoral artery, and the entry point now threatens to leak. This low-tech treatment involves applying almost thirty minutes of sustained physical pressure, doctor's fingertips to patient's flesh, over the incision to manually stave off massive blood loss.

As I remove my numb, stiff fingers, bleeding stopped, I've

completed my first year in fellowship, with apologies to T. S. Eliot, not with a bang but with a look back. . . .

I take inventory of what I think are the lessons of the year. First and foremost, fellowship is not heroic. It's not 365 days of testosterone. It's not war. The value is in the pure learning. In residency, the education can be something of a brutal rite, the medical equivalent of *One L,* Scott Turow's revealing look at law school. The process taxes you, overloads you, tests you—physically and mentally—demanding that you learn the basics of so many disciplines, fast, and under pressure.

Fellowship is hard in an almost opposite way: all about focus—intense focus. We learn a great deal about one thing—cardiology and each of its facets, but all still cardiology. It's not an endurance test. It's a chess game, taking in the whole picture, seeing where danger lurks, finding paths through the maze, reckoning with the ramifications of each. If X happens, I do Y, but if Z happens, I absolutely do not do Y. Fellowship zeroes in on the subject and mines it, and leaves us with a greater depth of knowledge. It's analytical. It's distilled. It's pure.

Fellowship is solitary, to a large extent, up to the Fellow. The rotations are predetermined. The attendings are who they are. But once in a rotation, I have a lot of control over what I do each day and whom I learn from. I can skip over things that are a waste of time and immerse myself in the areas I like, and I can, for the most part, pick my mentors.

Fellowship, despite the literal meaning of the word, is not a team or group experience, not "we" as much as "me." When

I started, I thought the other Fellows would be my world, the people I'd live, breathe, eat, or stay up all night with discussing cases. That's more residency than fellowship. In fact, I hardly know the other Fellows. I know the attendings better because the learning has been one-on-one, me and an attending. I miss the collegial aspect, but the reality is, now it's not about how well you play or work with others; it's about making you as highly trained as possible in each particular skill.

But, as a result, after a full year of fellowship, because we work solo, I don't really know who, in my class, is a good doctor and who isn't. Unlike residency, there's no opportunity to see their performance, style, or knowledge, save the rare glimpses in case conferences.

Has fellowship made me a better doctor? In some ways yes, in others maybe, in still others the jury is out. I'm not smarter than I was a year ago, because, at this point in life, I don't think you suddenly get more intelligent. But I am better at what I do. I've seen and experienced a lot. And absorbed it. There's value in pattern recognition and in having mysteries demystified. It's about generating sufficient experiential data regarding certain things to be able to responsibly make decisions for patients. People say there is an important difference between intelligence and wisdom. Intelligence is limited. You go as far as you can go. Wisdom continues. I am hoping to get wiser.

Have I gained any wisdom? Am I wiser? The confluence of events that closed out the year—the end of preventive, part III of echo, and the groin hold—resonate with me more than any single rotation, procedure, doctor, or outcome. Too often we think medicine is about heroic dreamers chasing miracles such as Dr. Franklin's Don Quixote–like quest for extended life by way of prevention, or the futuristic but flawed wizardry of devices that purport to "read" the body and tell us just what is wrong and what to do. Then we get the sobering reality check that, for Ms. Bailey or the elderly woman who needed a literal human tourniquet on her groin or most people with most illnesses, for that matter, it's simple measures that heal, or try to, keeping patients alive another day. Medicine is not one, but all of these—lofty, technological, and primitive—although we often forget it.

It's an appropriate segue into my next endeavor. Rather than going straight into year two of fellowship, I've been asked to be a chief in the internal medicine residency program. At Hopkins, the chief year does not directly follow the completion of your own residency. Hopkins believes that the chief should perform the function after having gone on to a fellowship, or research, or into practice, to bring more perspective and experience to the job. It's physically far more taxing than fellowship, and adds another year to my endless training, but it's an honor and a teaching/learning/mentoring opportunity.

On Monday, when I begin, I'll take a page from Dr. Fitzgerald's welcome to fellowship, in which he noted something meaningful or distinguishing he'd gleaned from each of our backgrounds, by doing likewise with my new group of mentees. I hope to show them, as he did, that beyond GPAs or résumé credentials, their human individuality is of equal or greater importance in caring for people. I hope to bring them some wisdom.

EPILOGUE

What Kind of Heart Doctor Will I Be?

I have to make the hard decision. I've put it off as long as I could. Now . . . what kind of cardiologist will I be? My path took me through year one of my Hopkins fellowship, the chief resident year, and then the second year of the Hopkins fellowship. The following year, my wife, Kelly, also a cardiology fellow, and I moved to Duke, she for heart transplant experience, me for a year of clinical research. That was a big change—all study and no patient care, something I wasn't sure I'd like but ended up thriving on. The next year took us to Vanderbilt, with Kelly joining the heart transplant faculty and me completing the final fellowship year—a combination of clinical research and clinical work anchored in the CICU, with the ultimate goal of becoming an attending. One year later, I was named to the cardiology faculty of Vanderbilt.

After four years of med school, and residency, policy

school, and fellowship; after all the rotations, all the attendings, all the patients, all the hours, and all the experiences—
the fascinating and the mundane, the charismatic gurus and
high-tech geeks, patient interaction and laboratory solitude,
ICU drama and echo lab tedium, lives saved and lives beyond saving . . . after all of it, which did I choose? For now, a
combination. But surprisingly, one not dominated solely by
patient care, to which I have always felt a compelling bond,
but by a combination of patient care and research . . . with
the aim of delivering better care to more patients.

For me, it was as close to an aha moment as I've ever had.
When it came time to choose, I realized the "how" behind
making people better drives me as much as the "doing." Beyond lowering one fever at a time, setting one fracture, or
even restarting a heart is the research—studies of correla-
tions and patterns of symptoms and living conditions, illness and lifestyle behaviors, laboratory discoveries that may
turn odds around, theories and conclusions that can impact
thousands, maybe millions, of patients at a time. As a physician, I want to make people well, but I want to make more
people well, as many as possible, faster. Like many of my
colleagues, I have an impatience with disease, an impatience
I hope will lead to changes and improvements in care. Maybe
the aha came as a result of my training, but as likely, it's also
in my genes—my grandparents' quietly demanding standards, my parents' predilection toward academics and research, my own study of public policy and politics, my
discomfort with healthcare inequality, a love of teaching . . .
all coming together and crystallizing at the moment of decision.

Today, I am an attending—a researcher who treats patients . . . and teaches. Not only did I find what I want, but I found a position in which to do it.

My job is split between clinical research and patient care. My research focuses on how to improve healthcare through systems-based approaches. That's a very broad aim, and it takes several forms. One aspect is about improving outcomes by getting people to the hospital—to the point of treatment—more efficiently. For example, if someone has a heart attack, the sooner that person gets to the hospital and into the cath lab, and gets a closed artery opened up, the better the person's chance of survival. But it isn't just a matter of dispatching an ambulance more quickly or having the ambulance driver's GPS avoid traffic, though those things help. It involves myriad factors interacting to optimize the process: Transporting patients via ambulances versus helicopters (helicopters are faster but because of availability and deployment delays, not always the fastest means of transport), plus "decisioning" software that can help make that call. Transmitting key data from EMS teams in the field to receiving hospitals. Delivering treatments to patients in the field before they even get to hospitals. Improving ER throughput, or how efficiently a patient is logged in and treated once there, and how to shorten that time. It's about every minute a patient is not treated and how to eliminate those minutes, about coordinating all these factors.

I'm doing this work along with a group of like-minded colleagues, experts at Vanderbilt, collaborators at Duke, and others with national expertise. Our goals are aimed not only at getting people to treatment faster but also at unclogging the treatment process, getting less-sick people out of the way of the more sick. I'm part of a team submitting a research grant application to the National Institutes of Health. Every year, 7 million people present to an ER with chest pain. Some are having heart attacks; some have the risk of heart attack; and 1.5 million have similar symptoms but likely do not have cardiac issues at all, yet still get much if not all of the cardiac testing. Are there better ways to take care of the lower-risk patients, to identify them and get them safely out of the ER, in order to reach those at real risk faster, in time to save more lives? We think so, and we have specific ideas on how to do it. It would potentially be good for hospitals, good for healthcare costs, good for long-term health, and good for individual patients.

And that is where I am spending the rest of my time, in direct patient care, as an attending in the CICU and in my outpatient clinic. I treat patients who may or may not have heart disease, or just present with risk factors, some of which involves general cardiology, some preventive cardiology, some in the intensive care unit. I'm working with Fellows, residents, and sometimes med students. I teach to pass on what I know while working to fill the existing gaps in my own knowledge and understanding of disease (the process never ends). I treat because, at the most basic level, that's what people who are sick need most. Conversely, the clinical care that I provide, the time I spend at the bedside, is a vital ingredient in making my research efforts better, truer, and more real.

I think back to when I applied for the fellowship and looked around at my friends who were already out in the world, practicing their professions, earning a living, being adults, and wondered when and if this training would ever be over. Undergrad, medical school, master's, residency, fellowship, chief year, more fellowship, now research. . . . Is there always more? Yes. Does it ever end, the learning and training and practicing and teaching and experiences? No. But it is no longer discouraging. It's good. It's good for doctors and good for patients. If it ended, it would suggest we'd found the answers, or given in to disease. This is how we do what we do. I've found my place . . . for now.

Acknowledgments

DANIEL MUÑOZ:

As I hope this book has conveyed, there are many physicians who have influenced my personal development and my fondness for the practice of medicine. Naming them all is not practical, but a few stand out for the lasting impressions they have made and for their powerful examples of how to care for patients: Steven Schulman, David Thiemann, and Phil Buescher.

The individual who perhaps deserves my deepest thanks is my co-author. Jim has been an immeasurably patient teammate, coach, and mentor over the many years that it took to turn an idea into a finished product. He took hundreds of hours of our recorded conversations and turned them into what I think is a compelling, accessible narrative.

And despite the challenges inherent in the entire process, he remained positive and retained his ever-present sense of humor. On the basis of his titanic efforts, he deserves honorary degrees in cardiology and in patience.

I thank my family. Alvaro and Beatriz are the best parents (and grandparents) anyone could ever ask for. Thanks to my sister, Ana, who is younger in years but whose wisdom and perspective long ago cemented her status as my older sister. Finally, I thank Kelly—the most beautiful person I know—for being who she is and for being the reason I pinch myself every day.

JAMES M. DALE:

Above all, both Dan and I thank our literary agent, counselor, sounding board, and part-time shrink David Black (who kept me focused and positive even when I was inclined to be neither). Further thanks to the entire David Black Literary Agency, in particular Sarah Smith.

Thanks to Random House for wanting our book. And our gratitude to Mika Kasuga for reading and editing, and re-reading and re-editing, and relentlessly making the book better.

I also want to express my profound appreciation to my co-author, Dan Muñoz. He opened up his world, let me take notes on his life, his training, his cases, good days and bad, literally life and death on a daily basis. I've worked with other co-authors, but none more honest, open-minded, and dedicated to their chosen field. By way of Dan's unpretentious candor, readers can live the rite of passage of becoming a cardiologist.

I cannot leave out of the acknowledgments the crucial role of my son, Andy, and Dan's best friend. Without Andy to connect me to Dan and vice versa, there would be no book.

And there would be no book if not for my wife, Ellen, whose idea it was, and who has most of my good ideas and then generously passes them on to me.

About the Authors

DANIEL MUÑOZ, M.D., graduated from Princeton University with a degree in economics, working summers as an assistant in a neurosurgery lab and as an intern for Senator Edward Kennedy. During medical school at Johns Hopkins University, he took a one-year hiatus to earn a master's degree in public administration from the Kennedy School of Government at Harvard University. After earning his M.D., he was accepted as a resident in internal medicine at Hopkins, and later as one of nine fellows in the hospital's coveted cardiology fellowship program. After further training at the Duke Clinical Research Institute, he is now an attending cardiologist at Vanderbilt University Medical Center.

JAMES M. DALE is an author and marketing consultant whose work includes books, articles, radio, television, sports, technology, media relations, and marketing. He is the former president of international advertising agency W. B. Doner, and the co-founder of Richlin/Dale business advisory.

About the Type

This book was set in Minion, a 1990 Adobe Originals typeface by Robert Slimbach (b. 1956). Minion is inspired by classical, old-style typefaces of the late Renaissance, a period of elegant, beautiful, and highly readable type designs. Created primarily for text setting, Minion combines the aesthetic and functional qualities that make text type highly readable with the versatility of digital technology.